MANUAL OF
FUNDUS DISEASES

MANUAL OF FUNDUS DISEASES

OP Ahuja
(*Formerly* Professor in Retina Service and
Director, AMU Institute of Ophthalmology, Aligarh)
Ahuja Eye Center
Aligarh, Uttar Pradesh (India)

Anupam Ahuja
Head, Vitreo-retinal Unit
Ahuja Eye Center
Aligarh, Uttar Pradesh (India)

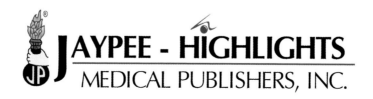

JAYPEE - HIGHLIGHTS
MEDICAL PUBLISHERS, INC.

Published by

Jitendar P Vij

Jaypee Brothers Medical Publishers (P) Ltd

Corporate Office

4838/24 Ansari Road, Daryaganj, **New Delhi** - 110002, India, Phone: +91-11-43574357, Fax: +91-11-43574314

Registered Office

B-3 EMCA House, 23/23B Ansari Road, Daryaganj, **New Delhi** - 110 002, India
Phones: +91-11-23272143, +91-11-23272703, +91-11-23282021
+91-11-23245672, Rel: +91-11-32558559, Fax: +91-11-23276490, +91-11-23245683
e-mail: jaypee@jaypeebrothers.com, Website: www.jaypeebrothers.com

Offices in India

❏ **Ahmedabad**, Phone: Rel: +91-79-32988717, e-mail: ahmedabad@jaypeebrothers.com
❏ **Bengaluru**, Phone: Rel: +91-80-32714073, e-mail: bangalore@jaypeebrothers.com
❏ **Chennai**, Phone: Rel: +91-44-32972089, e-mail: chennai@jaypeebrothers.com
❏ **Hyderabad**, Phone: Rel:+91-40-32940929, e-mail: hyderabad@jaypeebrothers.com
❏ **Kochi**, Phone: +91-484-2395740, e-mail: kochi@jaypeebrothers.com
❏ **Kolkata**, Phone: +91-33-22276415, e-mail: kolkata@jaypeebrothers.com
❏ **Lucknow**, Phone: +91-522-3040554, e-mail: lucknow@jaypeebrothers.com
❏ **Mumbai**, Phone: Rel: +91-22-32926896, e-mail: mumbai@jaypeebrothers.com
❏ **Nagpur**, Phone: Rel: +91-712-3245220, e-mail: nagpur@jaypeebrothers.com

Overseas Offices

❏ **North America Office, USA,** Ph: 001-636-6279734, e-mail: jaypee@jaypeebrothers.com, anjulav@jaypeebrothers.com
❏ **Central America Office, Panama City, Panama,** Ph: 001-507-317-0160, e-mail: cservice@jphmedical.com
     Website: www.jphmedical.com
❏ **Europe Office, UK,** Ph: +44 (0) 2031708910, e-mail: dholman@jpmedical.biz

Manual of Fundus Diseases

© 2010, Jaypee Brothers Medical Publishers

This book has been published in good faith that the material provided by authors is original. Every effort is made to ensure accuracy of material, but the publisher, printer and authors will not be held responsible for any inadvertent error(s). In case of any dispute, all legal matters are to be settled under Delhi jurisdiction only.

First Edition: **2010**

ISBN 978-81-8448-964-4

Typeset at JPBMP typesetting unit
Printed at Ajanta Offset & Packagings Ltd., New Delhi

To
Arjun and Aanchal

Preface

Fundus diseases constitute a major group of conditions leading to visual morbidity of serious nature, and blindness. As a result, it has engaged the attention of a large number of ophthalmologists allover the world. A huge amount of written material is available on various aspects of the subject. The present work is not meant to be a textbook or a reference book, but a kind of ready reckoner that may help the residents and busy practitioners in making the correct diagnosis and quickly refresh the facts about the basic aspects of the disease process, and understand the currently followed principles of treatment. It is hoped, the book will serve this purpose. The description of clinical features, as well as the treatment of various conditions have been updated.

In order to augment the visual impression of clinical picture of a disease, the book has been designed to include sufficient number of clinical photographs representing the disease in different forms of its manifestation. Wherever necessary, fluorescein angiograms have been included to explain certain subtle features of the disease process.

OP Ahuja
Anupam Ahuja

Acknowledgments

We are indebted to all our patients whose case histories and pictures have been utilized in the preparation of this book. Sincere thanks to our ophthalmologist wives, Prof Leela Ahuja and Dr Gayatri Ahuja for not only an overall cooperation and encouragement but also for the technical suggestions and constructive criticism. The support staff of the institution was very helpful.

Contents

Chapter 1: Diseases of the Macula 1

  1. Drusen 1

  2. Age-related macular degeneration (ARMD) 3

  3. Myopic maculopathy 16

  4. Macular hole 20

  5. Central serous retinopathy 22

  6. Retinal pigment epithelial detachment 34

  7. Cystoid macular edema 36

  8. Idiopathic polypoidal choroidal vasculopathy (IPCV) 39

  9. Parafoveal telangiectasia 41

10. Choroidal neovascular membrane (other than ARMD) 44

11. Choroidal folds 48

12. Choroidal rupture 48

13. Macular hemorrahage 50

14. Commotio retinae (Berlin's edema) 50

15. Epimacular membrane (EMM) 51

Chapter 2: Retinal Vascular Diseases 53

  1. Arterial occlusions 53

  2. Venous occlusions 58

  3. Hypertensive retinopathy 68

  4. Diabetic retinopathy 70

  5. Coats' disease 81

Chapter 3: Inflammations 83

  1. Acute multifocal posterior pigment epitheliopathy (AMPPE) 83

  2. Acute multifocal choroiditis 85

  3. Geographic helicoids peripapillary choroidopathy (GHPC) 86

  4. Toxoplasmic retinochoroiditis 89

  5. Eales' disease (Periphlebitis retinae) 90

  6. Sarcoidosis 94

Chapter 4: Hereditary Diseases 96

  1. Stargardt's macular dystrophy 96

  2. Bests' disease (Vitelliform degeneration) 97

  3. Cone dystrophy 98

  4. Retinitis pigmentosa 99

  5. Familial dominant drusen 103

  6. Central areolar choroidal dystrophy 103

Chapter 5: Optic Nerve Disorders **105**

   1. Myelinated nerve fibers 105

   2. Optic disk coloboma 106

   3. Optic disk pit 107

   4. Optic disk drusen 108

   5. Papilledema 109

   6. Optic neuritis 111

   7. Optic atrophy 113

   8. Avulsion of optic disk 115

Chapter 6: Tumors **116**

   1. Choroidal nevus 116

   2. Congenital hypertrophy of the retinal pigment epithelium (CHRPE) 117

   3. Capillary hemangioma 118

   4. Astrocytoma 120

   5. Melanocytoma 120

Chapter 7: Retinal Detachment **121**

Index *125*

Diseases of the Macula

1. DRUSEN

These are the yellow-white spots seen deep within the fundus, placed at the posterior pole in both eyes. Drusen result due to incorporation of amorphous, acellular material on the Bruch's membrane. Clinically, they are usually invisible before the middle age. The number of drusen tends to increase with age.

The function of retinal pigment epithelial (RPE) cells include structurally supporting and orienting the outer segments of the receptor cells, providing a nutritional interface between the receptors and the choroid, and regenerating photo pigments. The RPE cells also digest and recycle receptor outer segments by phagocytosis. The decomposition and recycling process of the RPE is quite efficient in young individuals but breaks down in some older persons. Hence, the breakdown products of the outer segments and other materials get deposited on the Bruch's membrane in the form of drusen.

Type of Drusen

Hard Drusen

Hard drusen are the smaller, discretely placed, round spots, sometimes with pigmented borders *(Figures 1.1A and B).* In majority of eyes, such drusen are innocuous and symptom free.

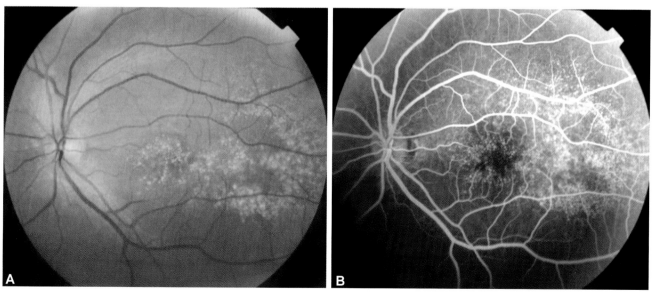

FIGURES 1.1A and B: Hard drusen
A. Pale-white, discrete spots placed at the posterior pole, in a cluster
B. Fluorescein angiogram shows numerous window defects, corresponding to the drusen.

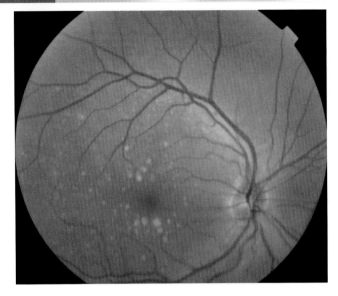

FIGURE 1.2: Soft drusen
The drusen are larger in size, with indistinct margins

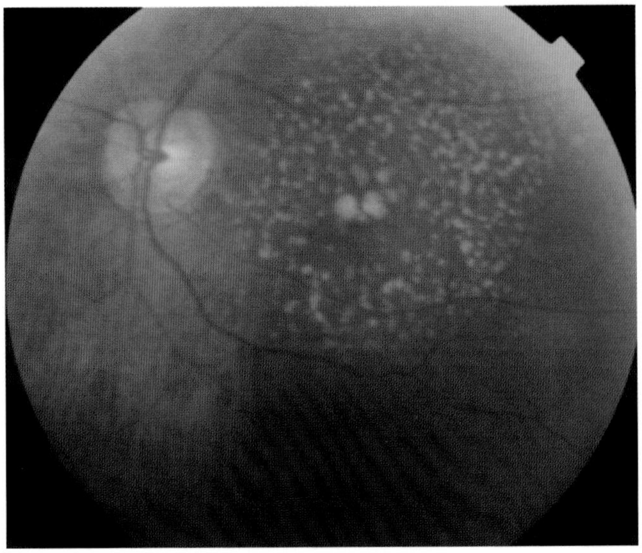

FIGURE 1.3: Soft drusen
Large, coalescing drusen

On *fundus fluorescein angiography*, multiple window defects corresponding to the atrophic RPE spots overlying drusen are seen in the choroidal and early arterial phase, and may persist in late phase due to staining.

Soft Drusen

Soft drusen are larger than hard drusen, and have indistinct margins *(Figure 1.2)*. With the time, they tend to enlarge and coalesce *(Figure 1.3)*. The prevelance and incidence of soft drusen increase steadily with age. In one study, prevelance of soft drusen increased from 7% among those aged 43-54 years to 44% among those aged 75 years or more. In contrast to hard drusen, soft drusen have been repeatedly associated with increased risk of the vision-threatening forms of macular degeneration. The atrophic changes in the overlying retinal pigment epithelium become diffuse. The risk of visual loss [dry age-related macular degeneration (ARMD)], and the development of choroidal neovascularization (CNV) increases (wet ARMD). The *fluorescein angiographic picture* shows larger window defects, fluorescing later than in the case of hard drusen *(Figure 1.4)*.

Basal Laminar Drusen

This condition manifests in the form of innumerable, subretinal round dots *(Figure 1.5)*.

Angiographically, innumerable dots of transmitted hyperfluorescence are visible throughout the posterior pole giving the appearance of 'starry-sky' *(Figure 1.6)*.

Treatment

No treatment is indicated unless the drusen are associated with a dry or wet ARMD. Trial with low intensity laser application observed that the procedure resulted in the reduction of the risk of advanced ARMD by 30% in high-risk eyes. However, Prophylactic Treatment of Age-Related Macular Degeneration Trial (PTAMD), in its latest report, observed no statistical difference in the treated and non-treated eyes, and does not recommend carrying out laser photocoagulation for the prevention of AMD in high-risk eyes.

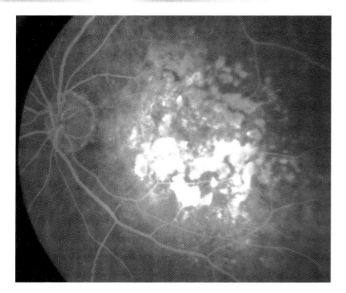

FIGURE 1.4: Soft drusen
Large window defects in the angiogram

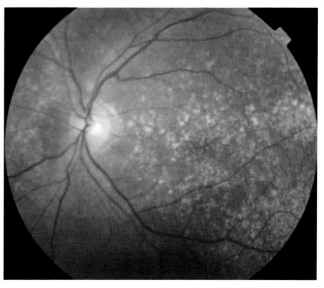

FIGURE 1.5: Laminar drusen
Large number of drusen seen throughout the fundus

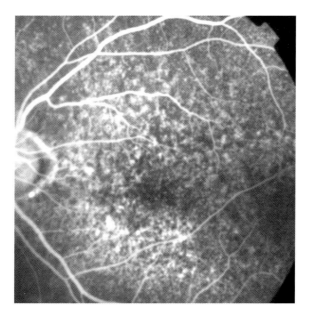

FIGURE 1.6: Laminar drusen
Innumerable window defects giving a 'starry night' appearance

2. AGE-RELATED MACULAR DEGENERATION (ARMD)

As the age advances, functional efficiency of retinal pigment epithelial (RPE) cells tends to decrease. Failure in the RPE cell degradation and recycling system, possibly occurring as free radical damage to molecules within the receptor outer segment, is possibly involved in the formation of drusen, the initial lesion leading up to the development of ARMD. Drusen are composed of photoreceptor outer segment waste products and other material that are deposited in the Bruch's membrane because of the inability of RPE to digest this material. If

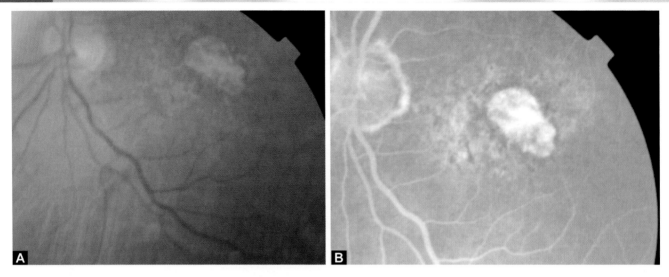

FIGURES 1.7A and B: Dry ARMD
A. A patch of atrophy of the RPE and the overlying retina at the macula
B. Large window defect at the macula resulting from the RPE atrophy

enough drusen accumulate in the membrane, exchange of nutrients between RPE cells and the adjacent choriocapillaries is compromised. As a result, the RPE cells die that leads to the death of photoreceptors, which derive their nutrition from the choriocapillaries via RPE cells. These degenerative changes at the macula, essentially because of aging, manifest clinically as Age-Related Macular Degeneration (ARMD). Two types of this condition have been described i.e. *Dry* and *Wet* type of ARMD.

Dry Type of ARMD

This is the most common form accounting for about 90% of all cases of ARMD, whereas the wet form is responsible for nearly 90% of severe vision loss. Drusen of the Bruch's membrane are the earliest manifestations of the disease. The risk factors include family history, aging, female gender (twice as common in females), systemic hypertension, smoking (increases risk of visual loss by 30-50%), light complexion and light-colored iridis, and hyperopia. As the pigment epithelium and the sensory retina overlying the drusen begin to atrophy over a period of years *(Figures 1.7 and 1.8)*, a mild-to-moderate decrease in visual acuity takes place. The initially small areas of atrophy gradually increase in size giving rise to circumscribed areas of RPE atrophy, focal pigmentation, and varying degrees of loss of the choriocapillaries *(Figures 1.9A and B)*.

Fluorescein fundus angiography shows multiple window defects in early cases because of the presence of drusen. Focal areas of hypofluorescence may be present due to the blockage of transmitted choroidal fluorescence by the pigment clumps *(Figure 1.8B)*. In the areas of geographic RPE atrophy, choriocapillaries fill slowly, or may be entirely absent in which case large choroidal vessels may become visible *(Figure 1.9B)*.

Treatment

No specific treatment is known. However, it has been reported that supplementing the diet of patients, who have a moderate or advanced dry ARMD, with anti-oxidants (vit C—500 mg; vit E—400 iu; beta-carotene—15 mg) and minerals (zinc oxide—80 mg; Copper as cupric oxide—2 mg) have 25% reduced risk of disease progression and decrease the risk of visual loss by 19%. The role of these agents in the prophylaxis of the disease is uncertain.

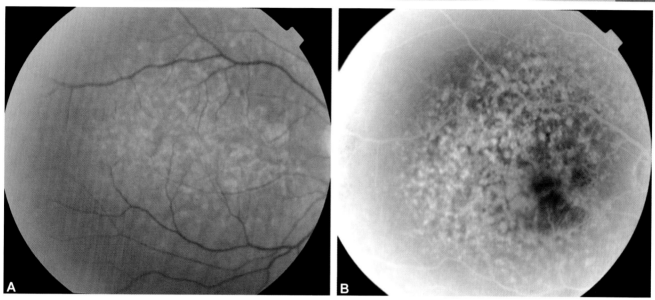

FIGURES 1.8A and B: Dry ARMD
A. A large zone of RPE atrophy
B. Hypofluorescence at the macula caused by atrophy of the choriocapillaries; large choroidal vessels are seen in the lower part of the lesion; spots of hyperfluorescence and hypofluorescence in the central fundus surrounding the macular lesion are caused by window defects over the drusen, and pigment clumping respectively

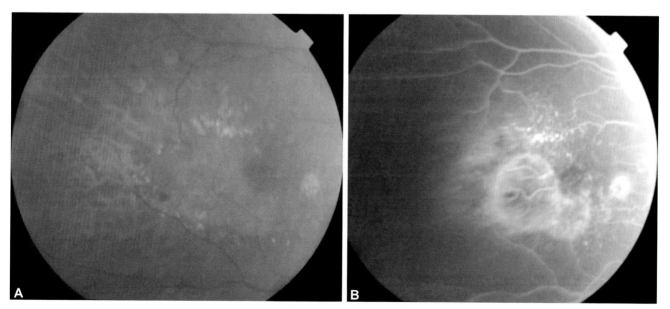

FIGURES 1.9A and B: Dry ARMD
A. Circumscribed zone of atrophy of the RPE and the choriocapillaries
B. Large choroidal vessels are visible caused by atrophy of the RPE and choriocapillaries

Supplementation of diet with 6 mg Lutein along with small amounts of vitamins A, C and E, zinc and copper is under study. However, it is cautioned that administration of Lutein to smokers increases the risk of lung cancer amongst them.

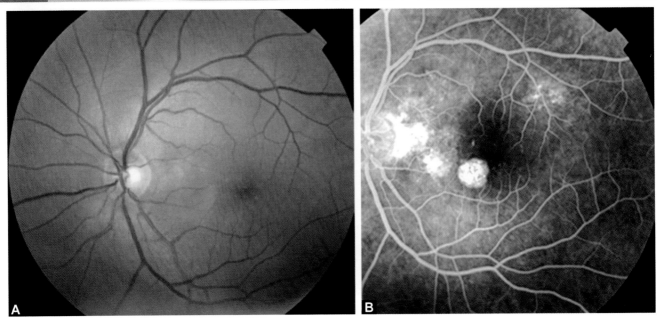

FIGURES 1.10A and B: Wet ARMD
A. Stage of PED, which is visible as a well demarcated, round area below the macula, and a
grayish zone temporal to the optic disk
B. Angiogram shows hyperfluorescence (window defects) corresponding to the location of PED. Spots of intense
hyperfluorescence within the PED are caused by the staining of drusen in the overlying retina

Controlled trials have been conducted to investigate the efficacy of laser coagulation in eyes with large coalescing drusen as a prophylaxis against the development of choroidal neovascularization. Although the procedure was effective in causing resolution of drusen, it was accompanied by an increased incidence of choroidal vascularization, both the phenomenon being directly proportional to the intensity of the laser burns. Trial with low intensity laser application observed to reduce the risk of advanced ARMD by 30% in high-risk eyes. Prophylactic Treatment of Age-Related Macular Degeneration Trial (PTAMD), in its latest report, described no statistical difference in the treated and non-treated eyes, and does not rcommend to carry out laser photocoagulation for the prevention of AMD in high-risk eyes.

Rheophoresis is another modality of prophylactic treatment tried in dry ARMD. Blood is removed from the patient, red blood cells (RBCs) are separated from plasma; plasma undergoes filtration to remove high molecular weight proteins (lipoproteins) and free radicals. The plasma is recombined with RBC and returned to the patient. Preliminary data show that 30% patients had visual improvement of more than 3 lines on ETDRS chart against the figure of 5% in untreated patients. However, the treatment has to be repeated frequently and indefinitely.

Wet Type of ARMD

This type of lesion is characterized by the development of choroidal neo-vascularization (CNV) between the Bruch's membrane and retinal pigment epithelium (RPE), or between RPE and the sensory retina. Drusen of the Bruch's membrane are the harbingers of choroidal neovascularization. It is responsible for 90% of severe visual loss related to ARMD. Subfoveal lesions, however, do not result in loss of ambulatory vision. The natural history of CNV never results in total blindness.

It begins with a serous elevation of the retinal pigment epithelium. Clinical picture of RPE detachment may be confusing unless examined with binocular visualization techniques. It appears as a sharply demarcated elevation that looks darker (unlike CSR) due to elevation of the pigmented cells of the RPE *(Figures 1.10A and B).*

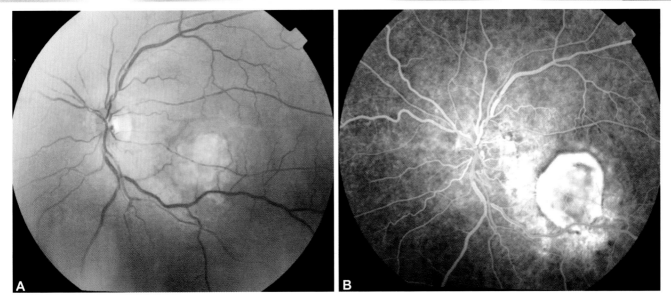

FIGURES 1.11A and B: Disciform degeneration
A. Organizing fibrous tissue caused by the hemorrhage from the choroidal neovascularization
B. Hyperfluorescence at the macular region resulting from staining of the fibrous tissue in the late phase angiogram

The RPE detachments may remain stable for several months but usually progress to a serous detachment of the sensory retina. New vessels arising from the choriocapillaries may invade the sub-epithelial or the sub-retinal space, with subsequent hemorrhage. Hemorrhages, thus caused, almost invariably lead to the formation of organized scar tissue, often referred as *disciform degeneration of macula (Figures 1.11A and B)*.

Patients with wet ARMD may complain of decreased central vision, central or para-central relative or absolute scotomas, central light flashes or flickering, impaired color vision, distorted vision (metamorphopsia), and prolonged recovery from light stress.

Fundus examination is best performed with slit lamp and a fundus contact lens or 90 D lens. It reveals gray or ill-defined subretinal membrane *(Figure 1.12)* that may lie in the subfoveal, juxtafoveal, extrafoveal, or in the peripapillary region. Subretinal hemorrhages are common and frequently outline the membrane *(Figure 1.13)*. In some cases, large choroidal hemorrhage may occur simulating melanoma. Exudates, serous fluid, or both are frequently present.

Fundus fluorescein angiography (FFA) is required in virtually all cases of CNV. Indocyanin green (ICG) angiography is required in some cases, especially for guiding the Photodynamic therapy. Optical coherence tomography (OCT) has become an essential part in the assessment of these cases. Confocal laser scanning-based imaging dramatically improves the image quality.

Angiographic Features

Angiographic features in a case of wet ARMD vary with the stage of the disease process as below:

Stage of RPE detachment shows a rapid and diffuse filling of the serous cavity in the choroidal and early arterial phase. The hyperfluorscence so produced becomes more intense during the peak phase. But there is no spread of hyperfluorescence. It remains within the circumscribed boundaries of the cavity, in the late phase *(Figures 1.14A and B)*. Unlike in cases of central serous retinopathy (CSR), it is exceptional to find a focal leakage of the dye.

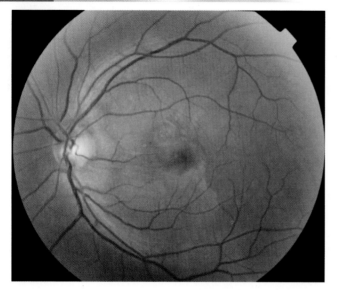

FIGURE 1.12: Wet ARMD
Gray looking, ill-defined membrane beneath the retina

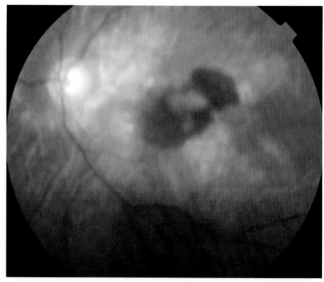

FIGURE 1.13: Wet ARMD
Retinal hemorrhage outlining the choroidal
neovascular membrane

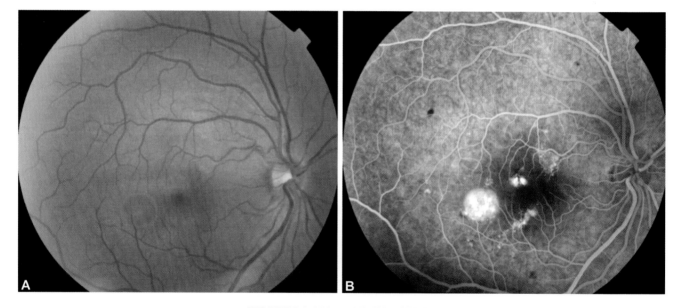

FIGURES 1.14A and B: Wet ARMD
A. PED (temporal to the macula) heralds the formation of choroidal neovascular membrane (superior part of the macula)
B. Hyperfluorescence contained within the boundaries of PED; juxtafoveal fluorescence with fuzzy borders caused by a small neovascular membrane

Stage of spontaneous resolution of RPE detachment manifests as a hyperfluorescence (window defect) in the early phase.

Stage of development of subchoroidal membrane (CNVM) exhibits two different patterns:
  (i) *Classic* CNVM, well-demarcated area of hyperfluorescence in the early phase. The intensity of fluorescence increases in the mid and late phases. The margins of the leaking area are well defined

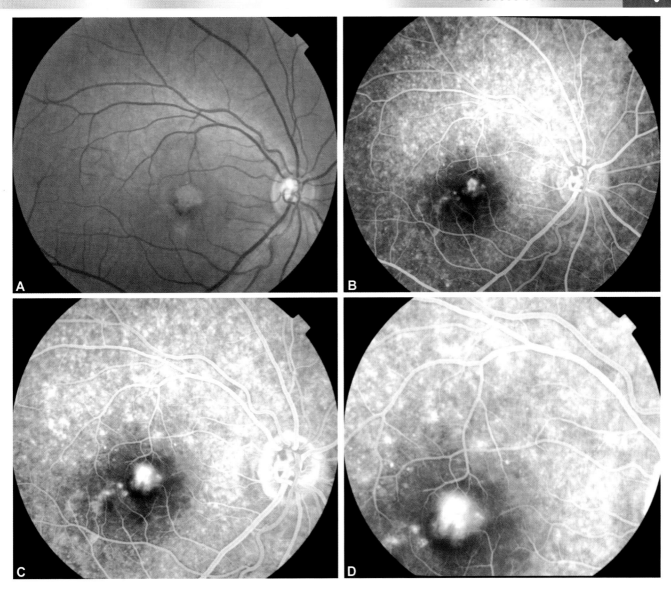

FIGURES 1.15A to D: Wet ARMD
A. Choroidal neovascular membrane
B to D. Serial angiogram of classic CNV shows hyperfluorescence with lacy pattern; hyperfluorescence
increasing in size with a spill-over beyond the margins of the membrane

showing a lacy pattern. In a late phase angiogram, however, the boundaries of the CNVM are obscured because of a progressive leakage of the dye *(Figures 1.15A to D)*. According to the location of the membrane, it is termed as *extrafoveal, subfoveal, or juxtafoveal (Figures 1.16 to 1.19)*.

(ii) *Occult* CNVM includes two types of hyperfluorescent lesions:

(a) Fibrovascular pigment epithelial detachment, in which hyperfluorescence is visible 1-2 minutes after injection of the dye, and corresponds to the fibrovascular tissue associated with the CNVM. The margins of fluorescence may be well defined or poorly defined.

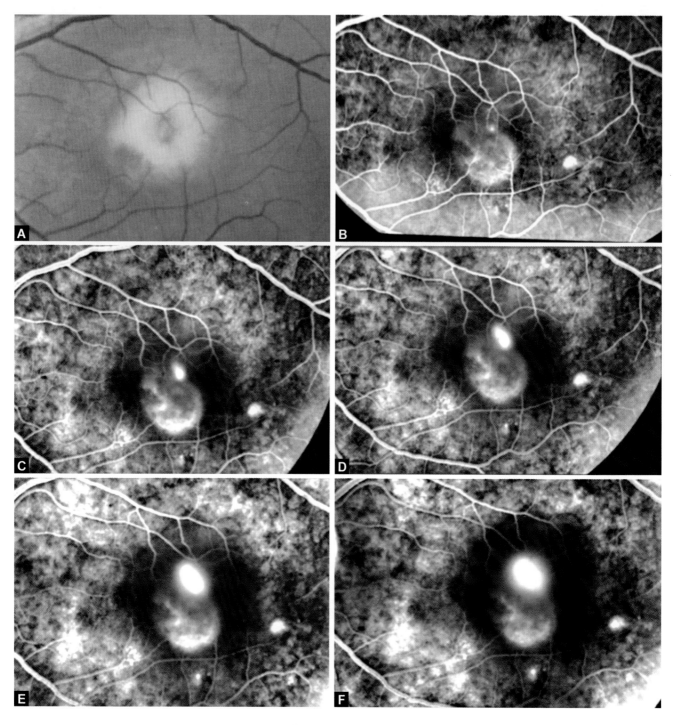

FIGURES 1.16A to F

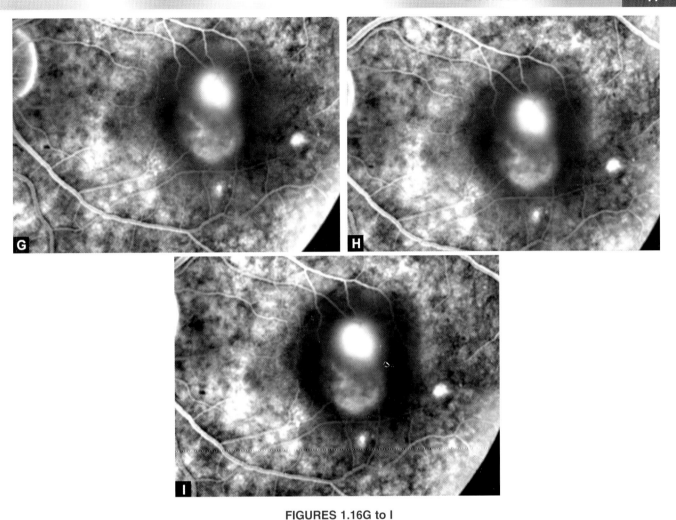

FIGURES 1.16G to I
FIGURES A to I: Wet ARMD
Classic subfoveal CNV at the margin of a well-demarcated zone of hyperfluorescence caused by PED

(b) Leakage of undetermined source, in which the leakage is seen in late and the source of leakage cannot be determined *(Figures 1.20A to F).*

Treatment

Treatment of CNV from the point of view of visual improvement is largely disappointing. Main aim of the treatment, therefore, is directed to possibly reduce the risk of further deterioration in visual acuity.

Various modalities of treatment available include argon laser photocoagulation, photodynamic therapy (PDT), transpapillary thermotherapy (TTT), subretinal surgery for macular translocation, intravitreal triamcinolone, intravitreal anti-VEGF and anti-angiogenic agents.

Argon laser coagulation provides a useful tool suitable only for classic membranes that are located in the extrafoveal zone. Macular photocoagulation of extrafoveal lesions has a 50% success rate, which is defined as preventing subfoveal extension of the CNV. Although Macular Photocoagulation Study (MPS) included patients with subfoveal CNV, these patients are no longer being treated because of an immediate loss of five lines of

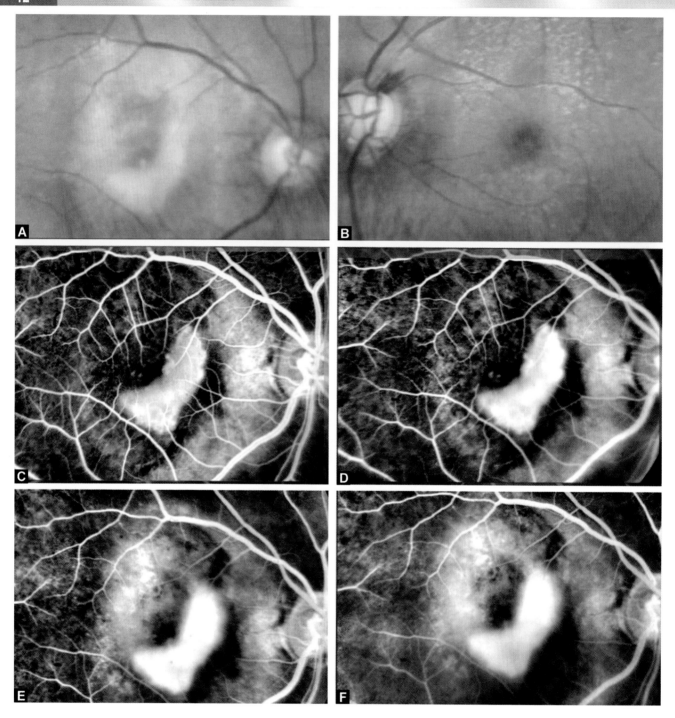

FIGURES 1.17A to F: Wet ARMD (Right eye)
Large juxtafoveal membrane

vision. Overall, about 13% patients with ARMD are believed to be eligible for laser treatment. Eyes with minimally classic or occult membranes, which constitute the major group of CNV, are ineligible for this procedure.

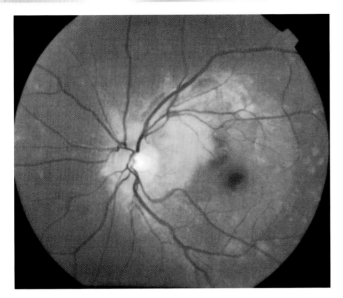

FIGURE 1.18: Wet ARMD
Juxtapapillary membrane

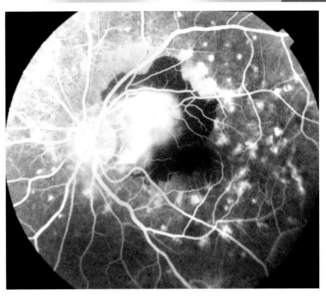

FIGURE 1.19: Wet ARMD
Angiogram of juxtapapillary membrane

Photodynamic therapy **(PDT)** is a two-step procedure. First, vertiporfin (Visuodyne), a photosensitizing drug is infused intravenously. It preferentially binds with the neovascular tissue in the choroid. In the second step, the retinal area overlying the membrane is exposed to a low intensity non-thermal laser. The laser light activates vertiporfin and kills the CNV cells.

PDT is particularly indicated in treating the classic subfoveal membranes but is unsuitable for minimally classic lesions. Photodynamic Therapy (PDT) study group patients with predominantly classic CNV were less likely (41% at 24 months) to have moderate loss of vision than patients who received Placebo (69% at 24 months). Patients with minimally classic CNV treated with PDT were not statistically different from controls. Lucentis has largely replaced PDT because of its availability since June 2006, and the widespread off-label use of Avastin since July 2005.

Transpupillary thermotherapy (TTT) uses a broad beam, long pulsed 810 nm infrared laser that penetrates beneath the level of retinal pigment epithelium. Clinical trials have shown that approximately 8-20% of treated patients had some recovery in acuity, 70% remained stable, and 10-20% continued to have declining vision. These results are far better than the natural course of occult CNV in which only 38% of eyes remained stable. However, the results of TTT4 CNV clinical trial showed that, at 2 years, TTT prevented moderate or severe loss of vision in 47% eyes compared to 43% control eyes, the difference being statistically insignificant.

Macular translocation. The procedure involves surgically moving or translocating the retina so that the CNV is no longer directly beneath the fovea. After the fovea has been translocated, the CNV can be treated with laser therapy thus, sparing the foveal neurosensory retina. Though an elegant procedure, complication of the surgery includes cyclodiplopia and the patient may have to undergo muscle surgery to correct the condition. Moreover, it is important to keep in mind that untreated eyes with CNV never go completely blind, while this outcome is all too frequent following macular translocation surgery.

Anti-VEGF treatment. Vascular Endothelial Growth Factor (VEGF) is a powerful mediator of vascular permeability, an endothelial cell mitogen and angiogenic factor. In patients with CNV, higher levels of VEGF have been found in the vitreous cavity. Anti-VEGF drugs, therefore, target both angiogenesis and permeability. Anti-VEGF treatments consist of injecting into the vitreous cavity, pieces of immunoglobulins that bind the

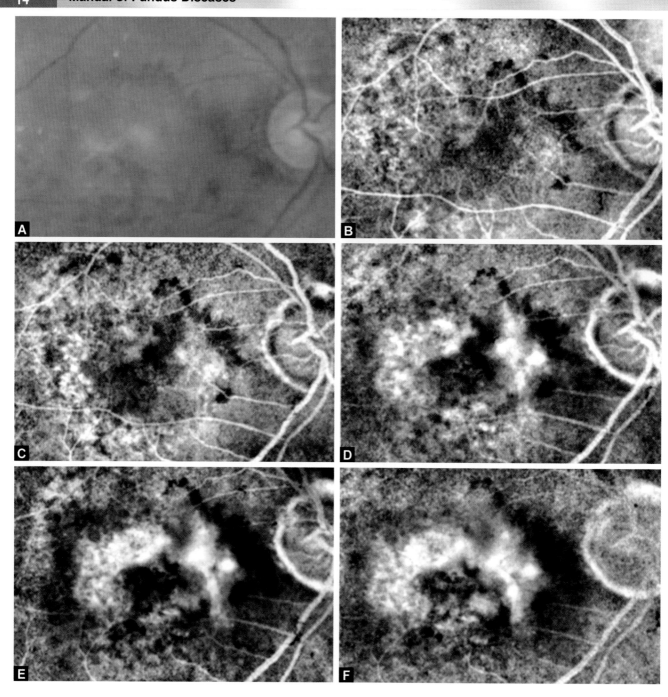

FIGURES 1.20A to F: Wet ARMD
Serial angiogram shows late appearance of hyperfluorescence with uncertain source of leakage—Occult CNV

VEGF. This inhibits its binding to the blood vessel endothelial cells and thus, inhibits the new growth. Beneficial effects have been observed, in controlled studies, with the intravitreal use of Macugen and Lucentis (both FDA approved) as well as with intravitreal Avastin (not approved by FDA for use in wet ARMD), in uncontrolled studies. The results are promising and show stabilization and suppression of CNV comparable to a degree similar to that provided by PDT.

Lucentis has set a new standard in the treatment of CNV because it is the first therapy proven to improve vision instead of simply slowing the decline in central vision loss. According to data from large Phase III clinical trials (MARINA and ANCHOR):

- Nearly all patients (approximately 95%) treated with Lucentis (0.5 mg) maintained (defined as the loss of 15 letters or less in visual acuity) and up to 40% improved (defined as the gain of 15 letters or more in visual acuity) vision at one year, as measured on the Early Treatment of Diabetic Retinopathy (ETDRS) chart.
- On average, patients treated with Lucentis in the MARINA study experienced improvement from baseline of 6.6 letters at two years compared to a loss of 14.5 letters in the Sham group.
- In the ANCHOR study, patients treated with Lucentis, on average, experienced a 10.7 letter gain from baseline at two years as compared to a loss of 9.8 letters in the photodynamic therapy (PDT) control group.
- Up to 40% patients treated with lucentis achieved vision of 20/40 or better.
- When Lucentis treatment was combined with PDT, FOCUS, a Phase I/II clinical trial revealed that 90% of the eyes treated with combined treatment maintained or improved their vision, compared to approximately 68% treated with PDT alone.

Following a report suggesting increased incidence of strokes in Lucentis treated patients, a large, randomized, Phase IIIb clinical trial-SAILOR (Safety Assessment Of Intravitreal Lucentis) was undertaken. The results of the trial indicate the drug is safe and not associated with a higher rate of stroke that had been reported.

Proposed mechanism of action of Lucentis is designed to bind and inhibit VEGF-A, a protein believed to be a powerful factor in the formation of new vessels. The treatment with Lucentis is contraindicated in patients having ocular or peri-ocular infections. The intravitreal injections may accompany, though rarely, by complications like endophthalmitis, retinal detachment, and iatrogenic cataract formation.

Current protocols for Lucentis treatment include:

- Assessment of all the patients with fundus fluorescein angiography (FFA).
- Patients have to have a sight 6/60 or better.
- Lucentis injection to be given monthly for 3 months.
- Retreatment if retinal thickness increases by 100 microns, as determined by optical coherence tomography (OCT).
- After three injections, a 1-month check; recheck intervals to increase if CNV inactive.
- PDT or intravitreal steroids may be required in some cases.
- Classic CNV responds much better.
- Occult CNV with pigment epithelial detachment responds the worst.

Macugen. This FDA-approved drug for use in the treatment of ARMD has been especially designed to bind and neutralize VEGF 165, hypothesized to be the predominant VEGF isomer associated with CNV in humans. The VEGF Inhibition Study in Ocular Neovascularization (VISION) comprising of two phase II-III, multicenter, randomized, controlled study observed that 70% of subjects, receiving 0.3 mg intravitreal injection every 6 weeks, lost less than 3 lines of vision versus 55% of control subjects receiving sham injections. The efficacy is similar to PDT treatment. Although the efficacy of mucogen is less than that of Lucentis, the drug is more effective when combined with PDT.

Avastin. Prior to the commercial availability of Lucentis, Avastin was attempted as an off-label VEGF inhibitor to control exudative AMD. Preliminary reports of intravitreal use of Avastin in ARMD were encouraging.

Systemic Avastin for Neovascular ARMD (SANA) study, an open label, uncontrolled pilot study with Avastin treatment (5 mg/kg of body weight) every 2 weeks for 2-3 injections, showed significant improvement in mean visual acuity and central retinal thickness. Numerous, small studies have subsequently supported the use of intravitreal Avastin by demonstrating decreased retinal thickness and improved visual acuity over baseline. Many ophthalmologists believe that Avastin is just as effective as Lucentis, but has to be given off label. Avastin is much cheaper (nearly 40 times) than Lucentis, both the drugs being made by the same company. However, all the research have been carried out with Lucentis. It is suspected that this is because the company has a conflict of interests, and there is much less profit to be made from Avastin.

A large, randomized, controlled trial to directly compare the safety and efficacy of Avastin and Lucentis in the Comparison of Age-Related Macular Degeneration Trial (CATT), has been recently initiated and the results are expected by the year 2011.

Anecortave acetate (Retaane). It functions as an anti-angiogenic agent, inhibiting blood vessel growth by decreasing extracellular protease expression and inhibiting endothelial cell migration. It has undergone trials to evaluate its ability to suppress CNV. The patients were treated with 15 mg of Anecortave delivered though a posterior subTenon injection and revealed 25% less loss of vision compared to placebo. When combined with PDT, 78% of eyes had no significant increase in visual loss compared to 67% treated with PDT alone. The FDA does not approve the drug.

Intravitreal triamcinolone suppresses the release of VEGF, lessens the inflammatory response caused by the CNV, and limits formation of disciform scarring. This form of treatment is especially applicable to minimally classic CNV that is not well defined on fluorescein angiography and currently not amenable to laser photocoagulation treatment. It causes a rise in intraocular pressure (IOP) in nearly half of the treated eyes, 2-4 months after the injection. In the vast majority of such eyes the IOP can be normalized by topical medication, and returns to normal values without medication about 6 months after the injection. Enhancement of cataract can take place. There is a report suggesting that depositing the drug in the subTenon's space posteriorly, is as effective as the intravitreal administration.

Lately, with the advent of VEGF inhibitors, treatment of ARMD with triamcinolone appears to have taken a back seat. However, in studies on combined treatment it has been reported that triamcinolone reduces the need for multiple sessions of PDT, prevents further visual loss, and improves visual acuity.

Squalamine It is a potent molecule with a unique, multifaceted mechanism of action that blocks the action of a number of angiogenic growth factors including VEGF, cytoskeleton, and integrin expression. The initial trials with squalamine in the treatment of ARMD demonstrated shrinkage in the size of CNV lesions associated with ARMD in some patients and stabilization of the lesions in others. In some of the patients treated with squalamine, visual improvement of three lines or greater was seen. Squalamine is administered intravenously, thus preventing the complications of intravitreal injections.

Among many other drugs in the pipeline, and at various stages of trials are Posurdex (intravitreal implant for dexamethasone release), Photrex (rostaporfin), ruboxistaurin (Arxxant) and Medidur (fluorocinolone acetonide).

3. MYOPIC MACULOPATHY

A progressive elongation of the eye (progressive or degenerative myopia) is accompanied by certain degenerative changes at the posterior pole of the eye that may seriously compromise the quality of central vision. It presents in the majority of people, as an inherited genetic condition and hence the incidence varies so much between different ethnic groups.

The degenerative changes vary in degree and extent, in different eyes. They include *Tesselated Fundus*, caused by the visualization of choroidal vasculature through the attenuated retinal pigment epithelium; *Islands of chorioretinal atrophy*, seen as white patches of visible sclera following the atrophy of the choroidal vasculature *(Figure 1.21)*; *Lacquer cracks* in the Bruch's membrane present in about 5% of eyes with degenerative myopia and manifest as criss-cross yellow lines at the posterior pole *(Figures 1.22A and B)*; *Choroidal neovascularization*

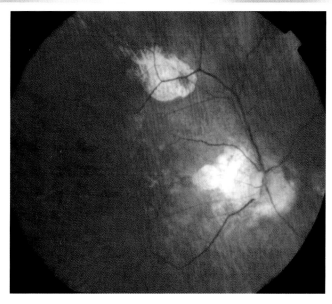

FIGURE 1.21: Myopia
Islands of white sclera visualized as the result of atrophy of the choroidal vasculature

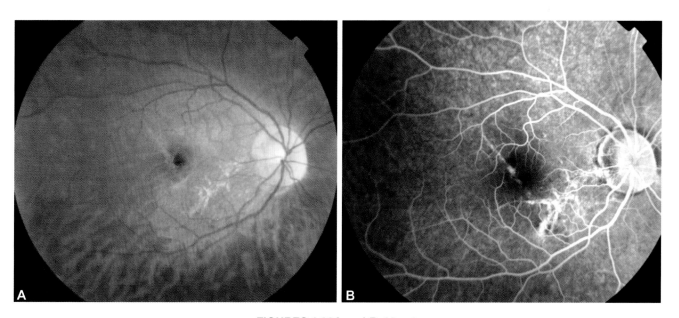

FIGURES 1.22A and B: Myopia
A. Lacquer cracks, visible as criss-cross yellow lines adjoining the optic disk on the temporal side
B. The cracks are better visualized in the angiogram

(CNV) due to development of vessels from the choriocapillaries under the RPE *(Figures 1.23A to F); Macular hemorrhage* with or without the presence of CNV *(Figures 1.24A and B);* and *Fuch's spot* that follows the absorption of macular hemorrhage with secondary proliferation of pigment *(Figure 1.25).*

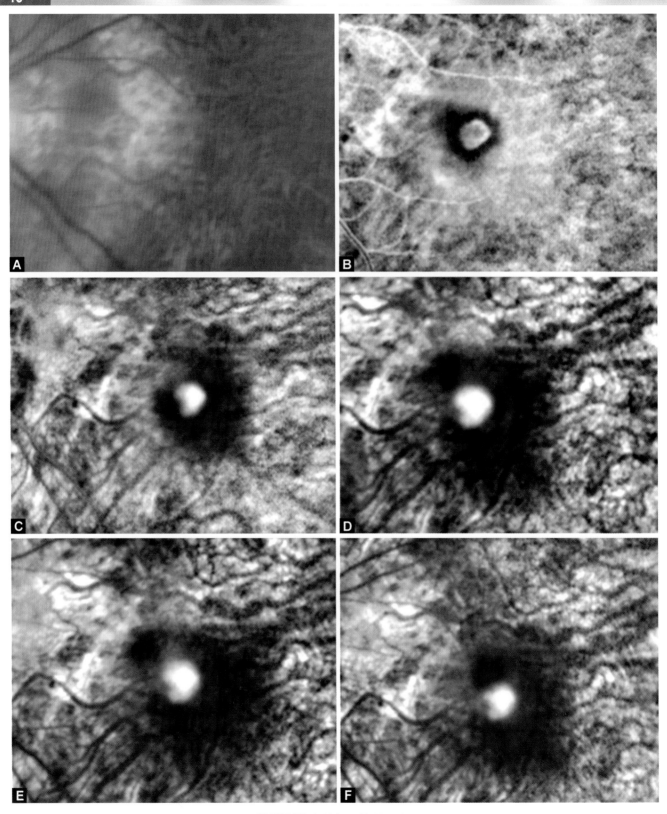

FIGURES 1.23A to F: Myopia
CNV in myopia

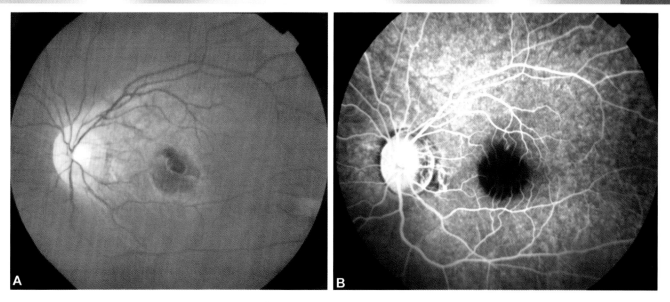

FIGURES 1.24A and B: Myopia
A. Macular hemorrhage in myopia
B. Angiogram shows hypofluorescence in the region of hemorrhage

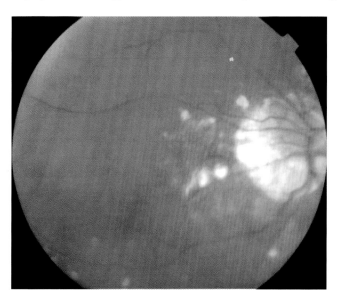

FIGURE 1.25: Myopia
Dark area over the macula following absorption of macular hemorrhage—Fuch's spot

Treatment

No treatment is known to cure or check the progress of the degenerative changes. Treatment of CNV, if present, is indicated.

Attempts have been made to control the progression of myopia by providing a support to the sclera at the posterior pole with the help of different materials notably, autologous fascia lata and donor sclera. Initial attempts in supporting the posterior scleral pole, that in retrospect, proved to be "too little and too late". In a recent controlled study, however, the procedure succeeded to stabilize myopia in the majority of the eyes under study.

Myopic macular degeneration worsens with both the passage of time and with the magnitude of the axial length of the eyeball, so that buckling adult eyes can stabilize axial length and perhaps, minimize future macular degeneration, but it cannot prevent the continuation of degenerative processes that are already at work.

4. MACULAR HOLE

This is a condition where a small piece of retina, partial or full thickness, dissolves from the macular area, under certain situations. It may be seen following trauma, solar retinopathy, high myopia, longstanding macular edema of any origin, or may be of idiopathic origin.

Idiopathic holes typically affect elderly females. There is a considerable, unilateral decrease in visual acuity. The patient may not be aware of decreased vision until an accidental discovery, on closing the sound eye for some or the other reason. The hole appears as a round punched out, red area with a rim of surrounding retinal detachment *(Figure 1.26)*. Multiple small, yellow dots may be visible within the hole *(Figures 1.27A and B)*. The other eye has a 12% chance of developing a macular hole. Complication in the form of retinal detachment is uncommon in the non-myopic and non-traumatized eyes with a macular hole.

Pathophysiology of the condition comprises of changes that take place at the level of vitreoretinal interface. The probable underlying factor is a focal shrinkage of the perifoveal vitreous cortex causing a tangential traction on the foveal area leading to foveal detachment and, subsequently, the formation of a hole. Based on this phenomenon, macular hole is graded into various stages as below:

Stage-1a: There is the appearance of a yellow spot, 100-200 micron in size resulting from the foveal detachment secondary to spontaneous longitudinal traction by the prefoveal vitreous traction.

Stage-1b (occult hole): The yellow spot is transformed into a doughnut-shaped ring of approximately 200-300 micron in size, centered at the fovea.

Stage-2. There is appearance of a full-thickness hole less than 400 micron in size. Spontaneous vitreofoveal separation may occur creating a semitransparent opacity, the pseudo-operculum *(Figure 1.28)*.

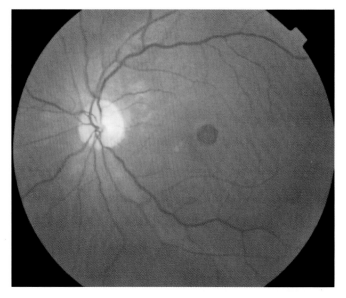

FIGURE 1.26: Macular hole
Round, punched out hole in the retina with a small zone of retinal elevation around it

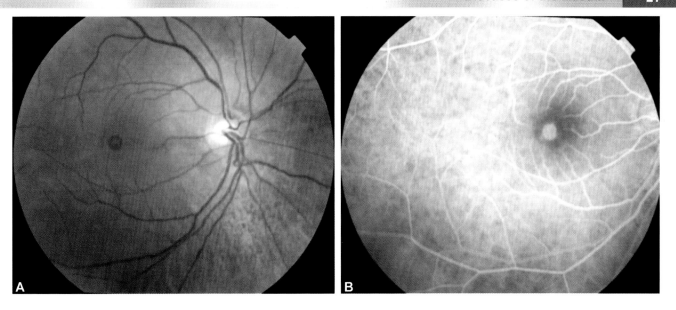

FIGURES 1.27A and B: Macular hole
A. Macular hole with yellow spots within
B. Hyperfluorescence corresponding to the hole

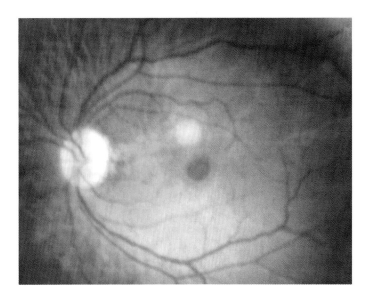

FIGURE 1.28: Macular hole
Macular hole with an operculum

Stage-3. The full-thickness hole is more than 400 micron in size and is associated with a partial vitreomacular separation.

Stage-4. The full-thickness hole is more than 400 micron in size but associated with a complete separation of vitreous from the macula and the optic disk.

Newer developments in retinal imaging technology, such as optical coherence tomography (OCT), give more information in the study of vitreoretinal interface and the formation of a macular hole. As a result, a new dimension has been added to the classification in the form of *Stage-0* macular hole. At this stage, there are no visible ophthalmoscopic abnormalities; but, the OCT imaging reveals that the fibers of the posterior vitreous cortex are still inserted at the foveal border causing an oblique traction.

Nearly 50% of Stages 0 and 1 holes do not progress and resolve both in anatomic changes and symptoms produced. Stage 2 holes progress and worsen, in 70% cases, to Stages 3 and 4 resulting in decline in vision.

A full-thickness hole has to be differentiated from a partial-thickness hole and a pseudohole. This is accomplished with the help of slit-lamp microscopy as described by Watzke and Allen.

Watzke-Allen technique consists of focusing a narrow beam of slit-lamp on the hole through a Goldmann's contact lens, and the patient is asked to report about the shape and continuity of the beam. In the case of full-thickness hole, the beam is broken, while it is unbroken in the case of a pseudohole. In the case of impending, small, or a partial-thickness hole, the beam is distorted, or intended on one or the other side.

Fluorescein angiographic presentation depends mainly, on the status of RPE. Full-thickness holes with alterations in the pigment epithelial layer *(Figure 1.27B)* shows increased transmission of choroidal fluorescence (hyperfluorescence). Lamellar holes with intact RPE appear dark, resembling the color of normal macula.

Treatment

No medical treatment is available. Vitreoretinal surgery may be indicated in full-thickness holes associated with a visual acuity worse than 6/18. The surgical procedure is addressed to the critical step of removing all premacular traction exerted by the posterior hyaloid, internal limiting membrane (ILM), and the epimacular membranes, if coexisting. The traction exerted by the posterior hyaloid on the macula is relieved either by removing only the perimacular vitreous or by combining it with the induction of a complete vitreous detachment. The removal of the premacular ILM is now recognized as an important contributory factor in the success of macular hole surgeries. The preretinal membranes if present are completely removed. A long-term internal temponade is provided using 12% perfluoropropane (C3 F8). Face down position is maintained for 2-4 weeks. Silicone oil temponade may be employed in patients who cannot tolerate head down position.

5. CENTRAL SEROUS RETINOPATHY

Also known as *central serous choroidopathy*, or *central serous chorioretinopathy*, the disease is characterized by a localized circular area of detachment of the sensory retina, usually over the macula that may or may not accompany detachment of the retinal pigment epithelium. Clinically, it appears as a blister like, round or oval elevation of the sensory retina of the macula, having glistening borders *(Figure 1.29)*. Occasionally, the lesion is located in extramacular retina *(Figure 1.30)*. The disease usually affects young or middle-aged person, often with a type-A personality (competitive drive, sense of urgency, aggressive nature, and hostile temperament). Males are affected 10 times more than females. The usual complaint is that of a relative positive scotoma and some drop in visual acuity. It resolves spontaneously in most cases within a period of 2-6 months. Recurrences and bilateral involvement may occur. On complete resolution, the visual acuity is restored, the scotoma disappears but the patient may continue to have some degree of micropsia, usually of little consequence, for a few weeks. Some permanent decrease of visual acuity may be seen in recurrent cases and in cases where the resolution of the condition is much delayed.

Fluorescein angiography is of help, particularly in making a definitive diagnosis in atypical cases, and to demonstrate, if present, RPE detachment, CNV, optic pit with serous macular detachment *(Figures 1.31A and B)*, and certain choroidal tumors.

Focal, dot-like hyperfluorescence begins in the early venous phase, increasing in intensity in the late venous phase along with leakage of dye spreading from the point of initial hyperfluorescence. Intense and enlarged fluorescence is visualized in the late phase.

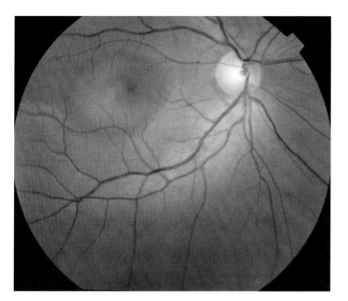

FIGURE 1.29: Central serous retinopathy
Circular zone of detachment of the sensory
retina over the macula

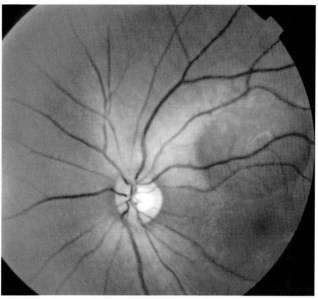

FIGURE 1.30: Central serous retinopathy
Extramacular location of CSR

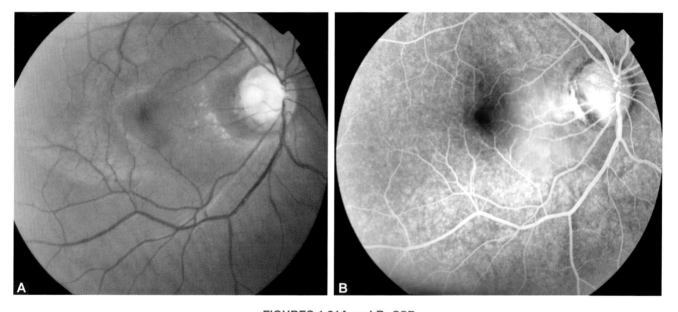

FIGURES 1.31A and B: CSR
A. Sensory detachment of the sensory retina in association with optic disk pit
B. Angiogram shows no evidence of dye leakage

The increase and spread of hyperfluorescence, caused by the leakage of dye from a discrete pigment epithelial defect, generally shows two patterns— smoke-stack or ink-blot pattern, the latter being the most common. An upward movement of the dye in a linear fashion produces the smoke-stack appearance until it reaches the upper border of the detachment. Thereafter, it extends side-ways along the borders of the detachment, assuming a mushroom-like appearance *(Figures 1.32A to I).* The ink-blot pattern starts with a point leak spreading in all

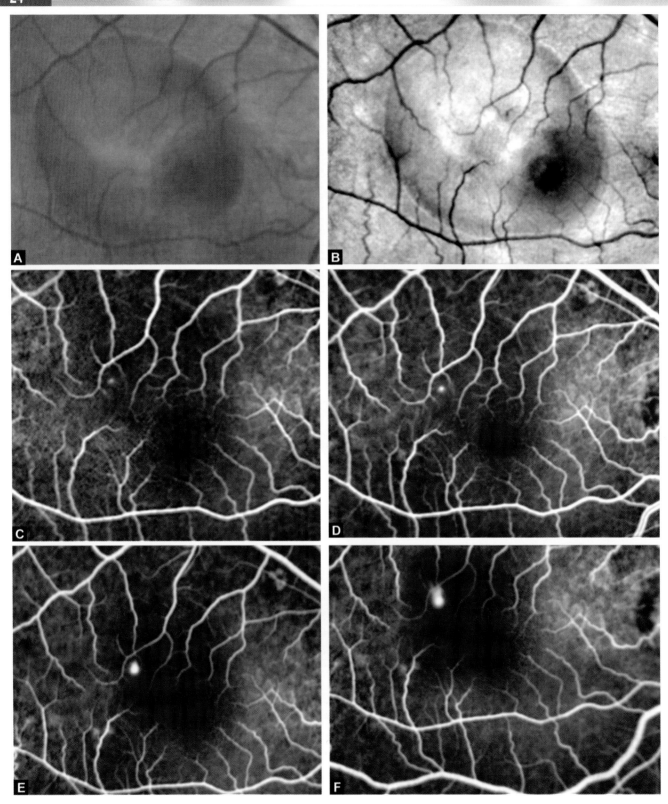

FIGURES 1.32A to F

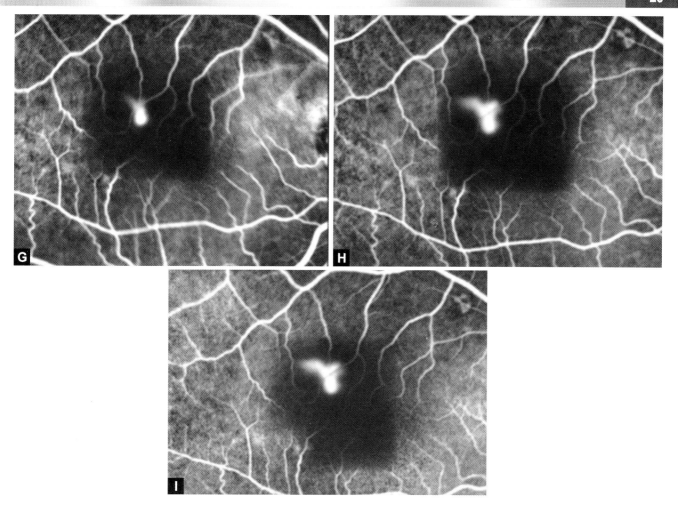

FIGURES 1.32G to I
FIGURES A to I: Central serous retinopathy
CSR with serial angiogram showing the progress of leaking dye to assume smoke-stack appearance.
Figure 1.32B depicts the appearance of CSR in red-free photography

directions of the subretinal space, but not filling it completely *(Figures 1.33A to I)*. Though usually single, multiple leaks may be present in the same eye showing either or both the patterns simultaneously *(Figures 1.34A to I)*. An absence of leak in the presence of detachment indicates the resolving stage of the disease *(Figures 1.35A to J)*.

Contrary to the angiographic picture of CSR, hyperfluorescence in pigment epithelial detachment, shows no increase in its extent in the latter phases *(Figures 1.36A to I)*. Likewise, CNV is distinguished from CSR by the earlier appearance of hyperfluorescence, occasional visualization of the capillaries, its lace-like pattern and diffusion of the dye all around its location *(Figures 1.37A to I)*. In cases of CSR associated with hemorrhage, corresponding area shows blocked fluorescence *(Figures 1.38A and B)*.

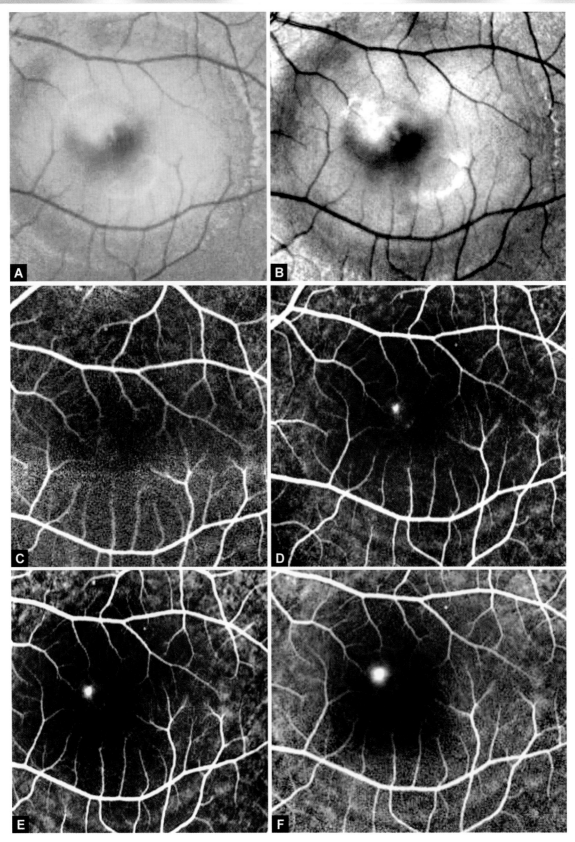

FIGURES 1.33A to F

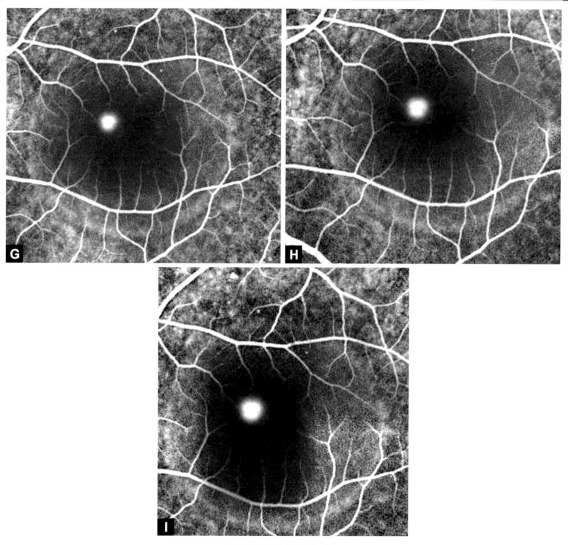

FIGURES 1.33G to I
FIGURES A to I: Central serous retinopathy
Formation of ink-blot leakage of dye in CSR

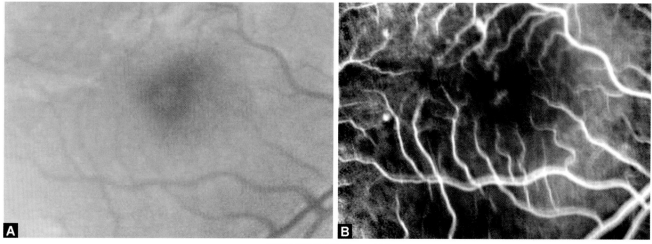

FIGURES 1.34A and B

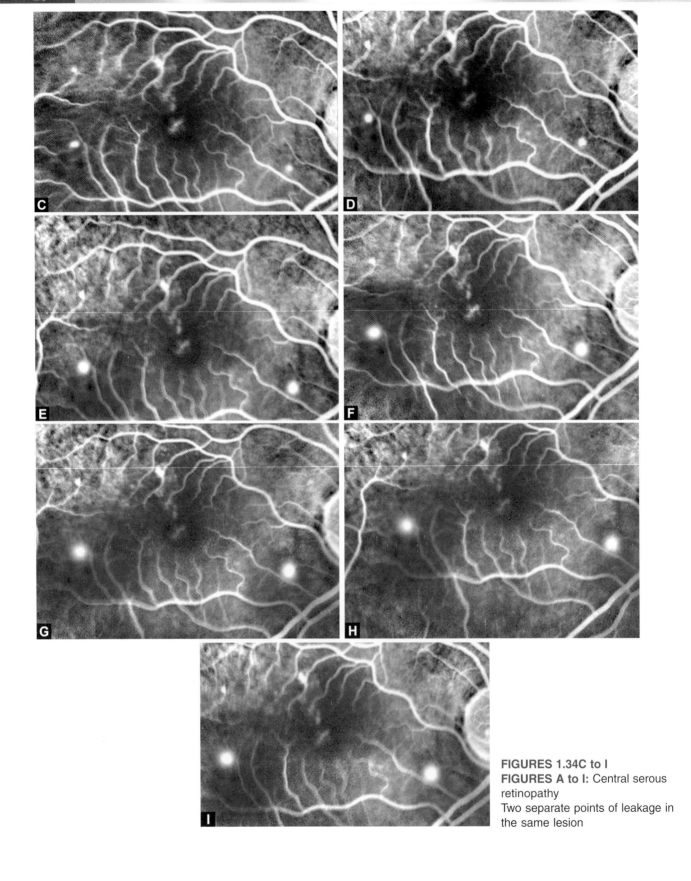

FIGURES 1.34C to I
FIGURES A to I: Central serous
retinopathy
Two separate points of leakage in
the same lesion

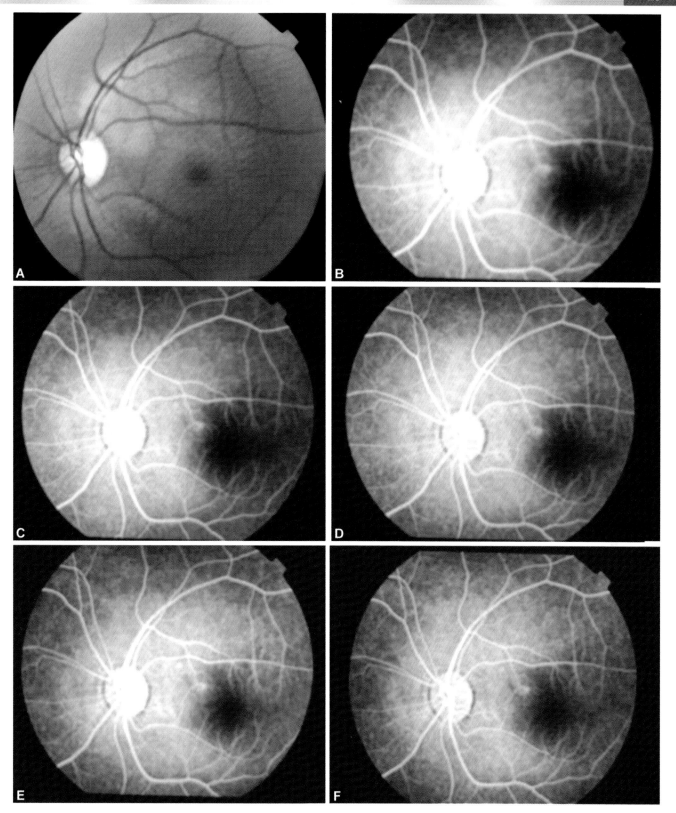

FIGURES 1.35A to F

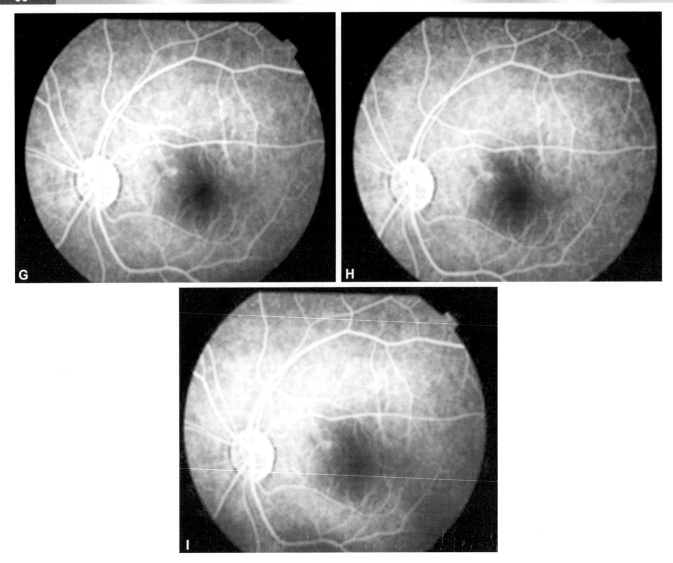

FIGURES 1.35G to I
FIGURES A to I: Central serous retinopathy
A. A typical lesion of CSR
B to I. Serial angiogram shows no evidence of dye leakage. The dot-like hyprefluorescence
seen at the upper nasal margin of the avascular macular zone is a window defect

Treatment

It consists of mild laser applications directly over the area of origin of the leak as localized on fundus fluorescein angiography (if located more than ¼ disk diameters away from the fovea). The treatment, however, is indicated only in selected cases such as non-resolving detachments with the leak persisting for more than 6 months; certain professionals (like pilots) requiring an early, excellent stereopsis; simultaneous bilateral involvement (rare); or a significant residual visual damage following a similar but non-lasered lesion in the other eye.

PDT has been suggested to treat the eyes in which the origin of the leak is subfoveal or juxtafoveal.

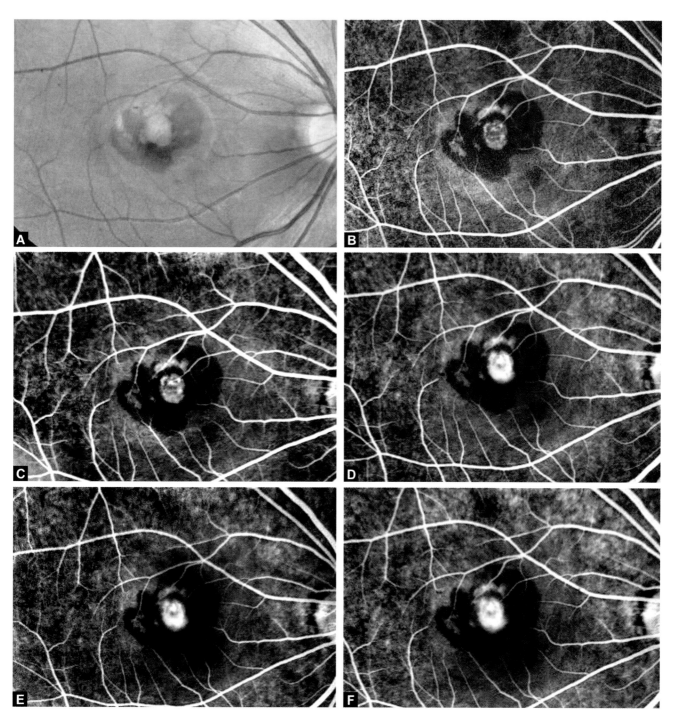

FIGURES 1.36A to F

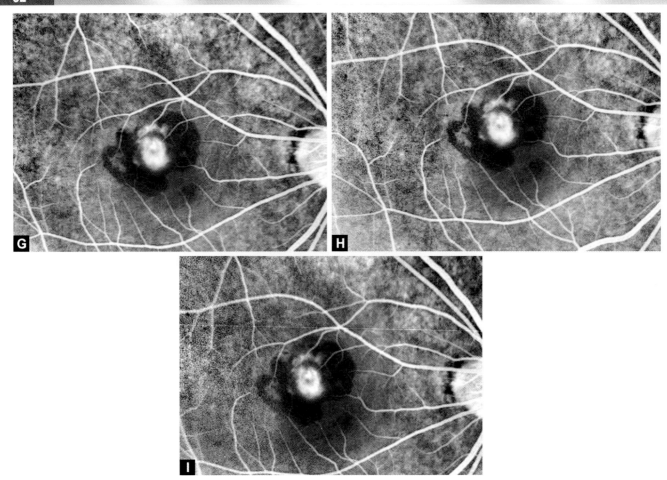

FIGURES 1.36G to I
FIGURES A to I: Pigment epithelial detachment
Serial angiogram shows a progressive increase in the intensity but not the size of the window defect, in the successive pictures. The surrounding hypofluorescence is caused by the choroidal hemorrhage—hemorrhagic PED

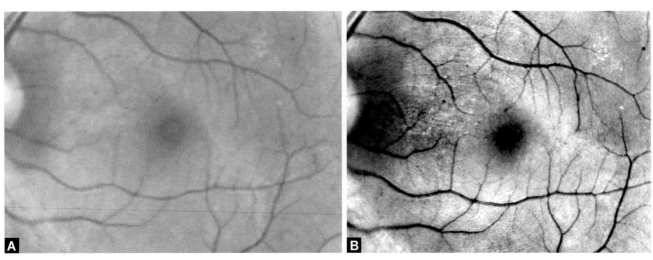

FIGURES 1.37A and B

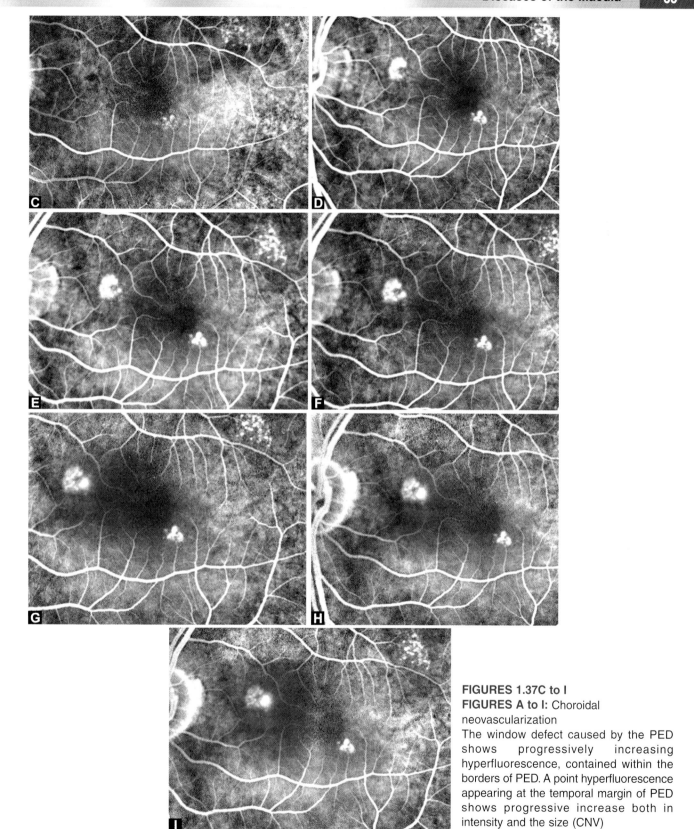

FIGURES 1.37C to I
FIGURES A to I: Choroidal
neovascularization
The window defect caused by the PED
shows progressively increasing
hyperfluorescence, contained within the
borders of PED. A point hyperfluorescence
appearing at the temporal margin of PED
shows progressive increase both in
intensity and the size (CNV)

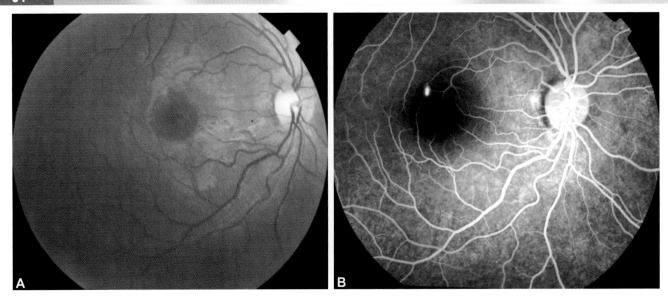

FIGURES 1.38A and B: Central serous retinopathy
A. A small CSR with hemorrhagic fluid B. Angiogram shows the leakage of dye in a linear fashion within the cavity of CSR along with surrounding hypofluorescence caused by the hemorrhagic fluid—hemorrhagic CSR

6. RETINAL PIGMENT EPITHELIAL DETACHMENT

Normally, the RPE-Bruch's membrane complex forms a compact membrane without a potential space between them. However, under certain circumstances, the normal junction between the basement membrane of the RPE and the inner collagenous layer of the Bruch's membrane may get disturbed resulting in the collection of serous (or sometimes, hemorrhagic) fluid between the two layers causing an elevation (detachment) of the retinal pigment epithelium. It is, thus, a non-specific anatomical alteration that may result from a variety of choroidal disorders like ARMD, choroidal neovascular membrane, high myopia, angioid streaks, hereditary choroidal degeneration, presumed histoplasmosis syndrome (POHS), and tumors of the choroids. Idiopathic RPE detachments are sometimes associated with central serous retinopathy (CSR).

Clinically, it appears as a small dome-like elevated area with yellowish or grayish discoloration *(Figures 1.39A and B)*. Occasionally, RPE detachment may involve a large area *(Figures 1.40A to F)*. It is best visualized with the binocular techniques of fundus examination. A single or multiple detachments may be present. The RPE detachments are usually small, less than the disk diameter. It may remain stable for several months followed by a spontaneous resolution without any residua or with atrophy of the cells. In cases undergoing a break-down of the outer blood-retinal barrier, serous fluid seeps under the sensory retina through the RPE presenting the picture of central serous retinopathy. Small capillaries arising from the short posterior ciliary arteries may invade the subpigment epithelial or the subretinal space—the *choroidal neovascular membrane* (CNV). The vessels in the membrane may bleed causing hemorrhagic detachment of the retinal pigment epithelium. Organization of the accumulated blood leads to the clinical picture of *disciform degeneration*.

Most patients under the age of 55 years who present with a small detachment without any other choroidal or retinal disease have excellent prognosis, particularly so if the detachment is off the foveal zone. Older patients of RPE detachment without the angiographic evidence of choroidal vascularization have 25-30% chance of developing CNV during their lifetime. Such cases need a careful follow up as well as home monitoring with the help of Amsler grid. Approximately 90% of cases with RPE detachment will manifest a concurrent serous retinal detachment, over the natural history of the condition.

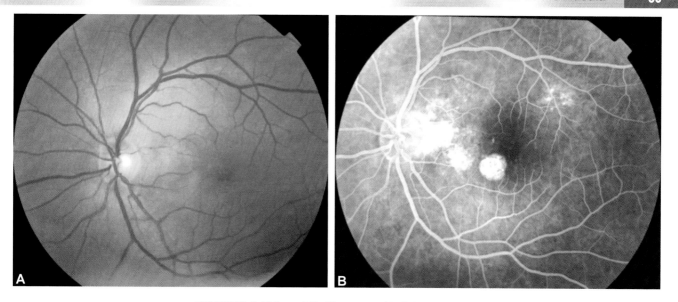

FIGURES 1.39A and B: Pigment epithelial detachment
A. A round darkish patch of PED below the macula
B. The late phase angiogram shows corresponding window defect. The hyperfluorescence caused by
the window defect is confined within the borders of PED

Although RPE detachment presents a characteristic picture, some other conditions like CSR, malignant melanoma, choroidal hemangioma, and Best's disease may have to be excluded in case of any doubt.

Fluorescein angiographic picture (Figures 1.40A to F) is characterized by an early appearance of hyperfluorescence in the choroidal phase within the area of detachment (rarely, a mild hypofluorescence may be present at this stage if the accumulated fluid is turbid). The intensity of hyperfluorescence increases in the arterovenous phase. The late phase shows an intense hyperfluorescence with sharp borders, i.e. the dye being contained within the area of detachment by the intact blood-retinal barrier beyond the margins of RPE detachment.

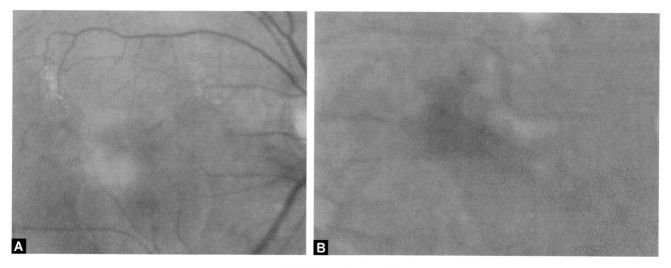

FIGURES 1.40A and B

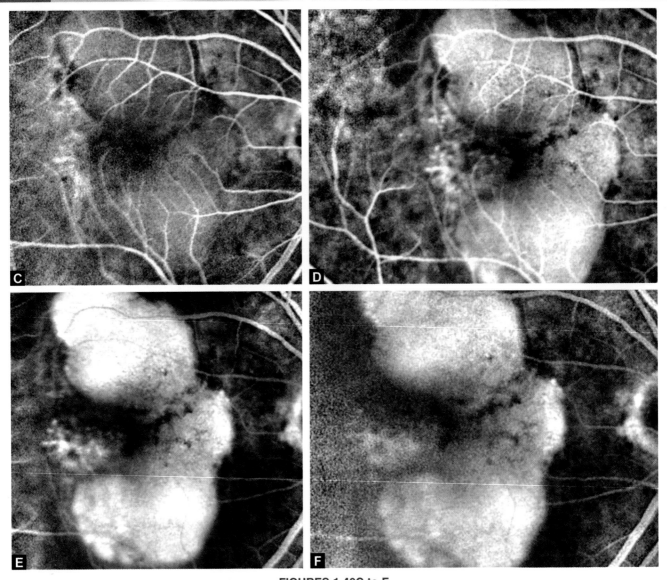

FIGURES 1.40C to F
FIGURES A to F: Pigment epithelial detachment
An unusually large patch of PED around the macula in right eye. The serial angiogram shows increasing intensity in the hyperfluorescence without a spill-over beyond the borders of PED

Treatment

Spontaneous resolution of pigment epithelial detachment (PED) without any serious residua is known. The treatment is directed at the management of the CNV, if associated with PED.

7. CYSTOID MACULAR EDEMA (CME)

It is not a specific disease as such, but the result of the response of perimacular capillaries to a variety of different conditions where leaking perifoveal capillaries lead to the thickening and edema of the macular retina. It is relatively a common condition related to ocular surgery (mainly cataract surgery), and other conditions like diabetes, retinal vein occlusions, chronic uveitis (pars planitis in particular), ARMD, choroidal

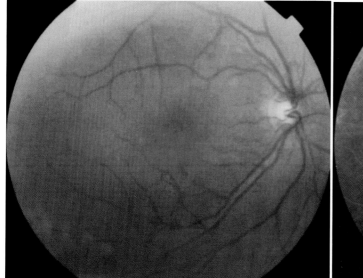

FIGURE 1.41: Cystoid macular edema
Loss of foveal reflex along with retinal thickening at the macula

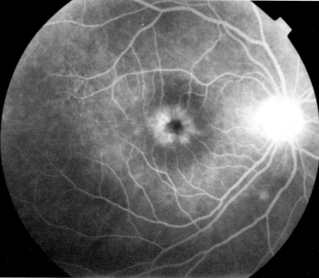

FIGURE 1.42: Cystoid macular edema
Angiogram showing flower-petal pattern of
hyperfluorescence at the macula

tumors, drug toxicity (prostaglandin analogs like latanprost), etc. CME of any etiology leads to significant visual loss. It typically presents with the complaint of a painless visual loss or distorted vision in one eye. It can be bilateral if associated with and caused by some systemic disease.

When CME develops following cataract surgery and its cause is believed to be directly related to the surgery, it is referred to as Irvine-Gass syndrome (also termed as pseudophakic CME). The more complicated the surgery (such as rupture of the capsule or vitreous loss), the greater the degree of CME and vision reduction. The retinal edema, perhaps, results from the release of prostaglandins in response to the surgical trauma. Prostaglandins cause a breakdown of the inner blood-retinal barrier leading to increased capillary permeability. Fluid collects in the loosely arranged outer plexiform layer of Henle, the fibers of which are arranged horizontally. This provides the basis for "flower petal" appearance of the lesion on fundus fluorescein angiography. Patients with postoperative CME has a 50% chance of developing it in the other eye. Beside cataract surgery, CME may also follow in some cases of penetrating keratoplasty, retinal surgery (pars plana vitrectomy), and YAG laser capsulotomy. The overall incidence of CME has been reduced to nearly 1% with the use of phacoemulsification techniques, as compared to 9% seen in older techniques like extracapsular cataract extraction (ECCE).

The condition is suspected because of the loss of foveal reflex along with thickening of the macular retina *(Figure 1.41)*. The diagnosis is made on clinical examination with the help of slit-lamp biomicroscopy of the posterior segment. Fundus fluorescein angiography shows leakage and pooling of the dye producing a typical "flower pattern" appearance *(Figure 1.42)*. Optical coherence tomography (OCT) demonstrates the cysts, but is especially helpful in monitoring the response to treatment.

Nearly 90% of eyes with Irvine-Gass syndrome show a spontaneous recovery but, chronic CME and frequent recurrences may result in photoreceptor damage at the macula and permanent impairment of central vision.

Fluorescein angiography shows focal hyperfluorescence in the arteriovenous phase on account of the leakage of dye from the perifoveal capillaries. The focal leakages merge into a 'flower pattern' *(Figures 1.43A to D)*, caused by the leakage of dye in the outer plexiform layer having a radial arrangement of its fibers around the fovea. A further spread of hyperfluorescence, if present, suggests a widespread capillary leakage.

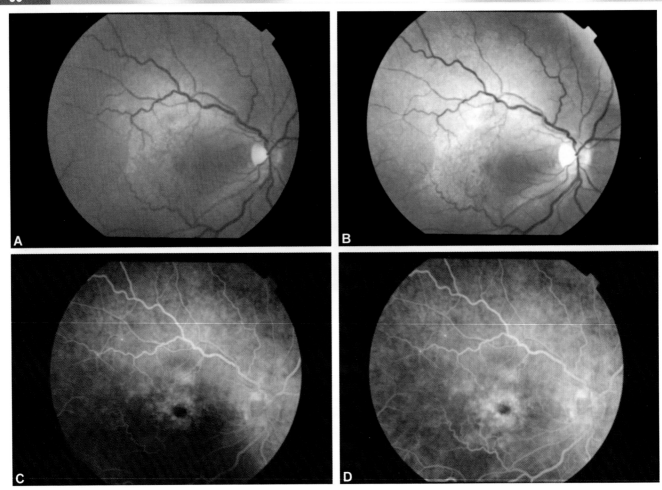

FIGURES 1.43A to D: Cystoid macular edema
The clinical photograph shows absent foveal reflex and retinal thickening of the macular retina that is better visualized in the red-free photograph B. The angiogram shows formation of flower-petal pattern of hyperfluorescence at the macula

Treatment

Treatment mainly revolves around topical or/and systemic administration of NSAIDs (like ketorolac, indomethacin, diclofenic, etc.) and corticosteroids. Intravitreal or posterior subTenon administration of triamcinolone acetonide shows good response in severe, non-resolving edema. Pars plana vitrectomy is performed to remove vitreous strands when tracking to the surgical wound although, YAG laser lysis of incarcerated vitreous strands is preferred by many.

Amongst the non-pseudophakic CME, diabetic macular edema is seen most frequently. Laser photocoagulation treatment is supposed to be a standard procedure in cases of diabetic macular edema. Site and nature of the leak(s) are established with the help of fluorescein angiography. Focal areas of leak are treated with coagulation of the areas of the leak(s)—focal laser treatment; while coagulations are placed in the form of a grid around the macula, in eyes showing diffuse leakage of dye. Significant visual improvement is uncommon; the goal of the treatment is to check progression. If the overall picture demands a pan-retinal photocoagulation (PRP), macular treatment should precede by at least 6 weeks.

Intravitreal injection of triamcinolone appears to hold a lot of promise in treating cystoid macular edema of diabetic origin. It has been observed to significantly reduce macular edema, and to improve vision particularly when the edema is pronounced. Action is maximal at 1 week, lasing 3-6 months. There is 30-40% risk of developing high intraocular pressure that can be controlled with topical treatment, in most cases; as well as 1% risk of progression of cataract, retinal detachment and endophthalmitis. Some have advocated it as the primary treatment while others consider it as an adjunct to laser photocoagulation.

Exciting possibilities are seen in the use of VEGF inhibitors in the treatment of diabetic retinopathy including macular edema. The FDA-approved drugs—pegatananib (Macugen), and ranibizumab (Lucentis) have undergone extensive trials in the treatment of wet ARMD, and have been found to be effective in regressing the disease process and improving the visual acuity. Bevacizumab (Avastin) is awaiting FDA approval (for use in wet ARMD) and has been found to be equally effective, as well as much cheaper. Available reports suggest these drugs to be effective in treating the diabetic macular edema, too.

Pars plana vitrectomy is advocated in selected cases of diffuse macular edema without having a posterior vitreous detachment (PVD). Vitrectomy with induced PVD may be effective in resolving diffuse macular edema and improving vision.

8. IDIOPATHIC POLYPOIDAL CHOROIDAL VASCULOPATHY (IPCV)

Also called *posterior uveal bleeding syndrome,* it is usually a unilateral, chronic disease characterized by remissions and relapses. It is found more commonly in the pigmented (Asian and African) races. It manifests in the form of orange-red subretinal nodules, representing polyps within the choroidal vasculature, seen usually at the posterior pole *(Figure 1.44).* Peripheral lesions may be present, occasionally. It is generally associated with hard deposits in the macula. There are repeated bouts of RPE detachments secondary to the serosanguinous leakage around the lesions. Complications are seen in the form of chronic atrophy, cystoid macular edema (CME), exudative maculopathy, and occasionally, sub-RPE or subretinal hemorrhage. Origin of the lesion lies in the inner choroidal plexus, and consists of network of choroidal vessels terminating into round, polyp-like lesions under the retina. Some consider the condition as a variation of subretinal vascularization rather than a separate entity.

At times, it needs to be differentiated from wet form of ARMD. Besides the disease occurring in younger age groups, fundus flourescein angiography and more importantly, indocyanin angiography helps to reach the correct diagnosis. Optical coherence tomography (OCT) may help in judging the stage (active or scarred) of the polypoidal lesions.

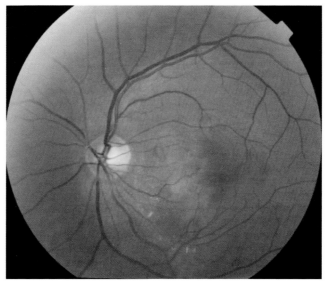

FIGURE 1.44: Idiopathic polypoidal choroidal vasculopathy
Orange-red patches at the posterior pole; some amount of exudation is present around the lesions

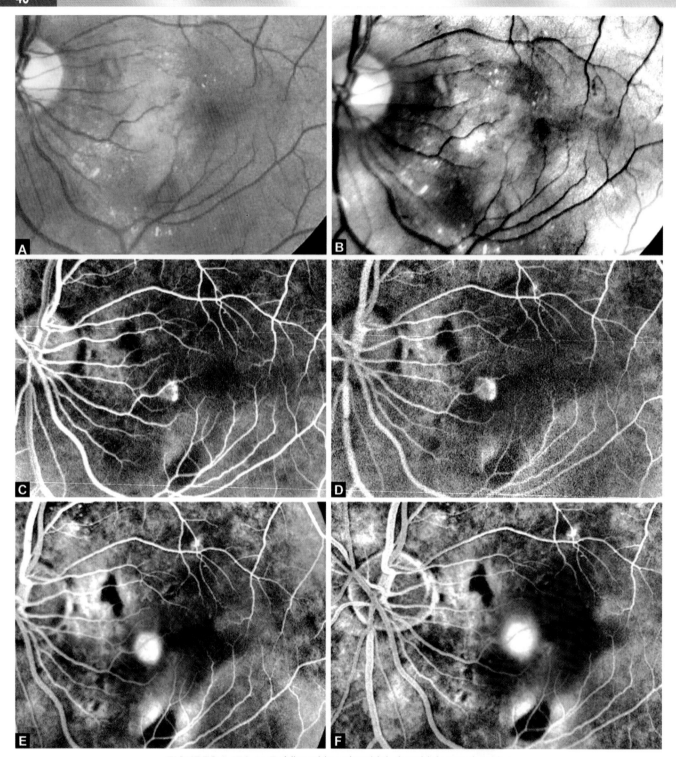

FIGURES 1.45A to F: Idiopathic polypoidal choroidal vasculopathy
Angiogram shows hyperfluorescence around the margins of the granulomas; hypofluorescence at the site of lesions is caused by subretinal hemorrhage; unusual complication is seen as hyperfluorescence that has progressively increased in intensity and size-CNV

Fluorescein angiography (Figures 1.45A to F) shows a stippled hyperfluorescence, from the areas of the lesions, in the early exposures. The hyperfluorescence increases gradually to fade away in the late phase.

Treatment

Treatment is indicated if there is a progressive exudation centrally. Thermal lasers or photodynamic therapy is directed at the leaking aneurysms, not at the entire lesion. Laser treatment targeting the feeder vessel supplying the IPCV lesions is considered to be safe and effective to improve visual acuity, especially in eyes with detachment of the sensory retina at or around the fovea. ICGA-guided laser photocoagulation can be considered as a modality of treatment. Subfoveal lesions may also be so treated. CME, if present, may be treated by injections of steroidal depots with variable results. Role of VEGF inhibitors is not known.

9. PARAFOVEAL TELANGIECTASIA (PFT)
SYN. IDIOPATHIC JUXTAFOVEOLAR RETINAL TELANGIECTASIA (JRT/JXT)

It belongs to the group of rare, idiopathic congenital vascular abnormalities in retina. Beside PFT, Leber's military aneurysms, and Coat's disease belong to this group. Telangiectatic retinal capillaries located temporal to the macula *(Figure 1.46)*, in one or both eyes, characterize PFT. It manifests as a slow vision loss beginning in adulthood. Most patients with bilateral disease have associated dilated capillaries, minimal exudation, retinal crystals, right angle venules, and retinal pigment hypertrophy. The unilateral form is not discovered until after the age of forty. Dilated and kinked vessels, along with microaneurysms in the foveal and parafoveal capillary network are the hallmark of the disease. Leakage may cause macular edema and reduced visual acuity. Fundus assessment reveals perifoveal dot and blot hemorrhages, and, rarely, exudates.

According to current convention, the disease is divided into three groups: *group-1* patients are predominantly male, telangiectasis is unilateral in most cases, and is readily visible. It is suspected that it may be a mild presentation of Coat's disease; *group-2* patients are characterized by juxtafoveal telangiectasis, minimal exudation, and right angle venules. As the disease progresses, intraretinal pigment plaques and subretinal vascularization may develop. In this group, telangiectasia is most likely caused by capillary diffusion abnormalities; *group-3* patients are diagnosed by bilateral, easily visible telangiectasis, minimal exudation, and capillary occlusion, which is believed to be the cause of the lesions in this group.

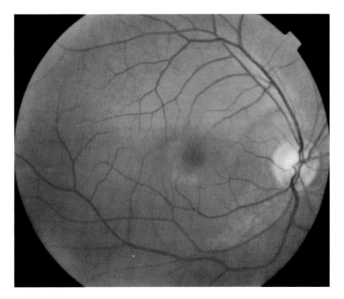

FIGURE 1.46: Parafoveal telangiectasia
A zone of retinal whitening temporal to the macula

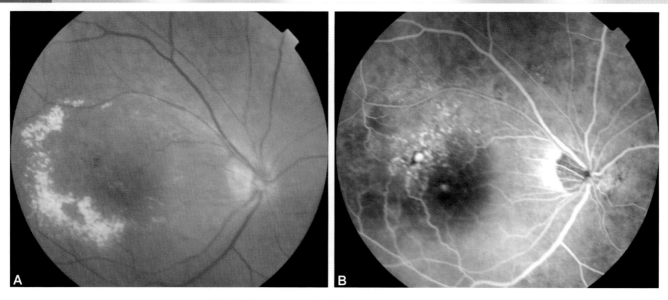

FIGURES 1.47A and B: Parafoveal telangiectasia
A. A girdle of exudates around the macula having capillary anomalies within
B. Angiogram shows hyperfluorescence from the telangiectatic capillaries

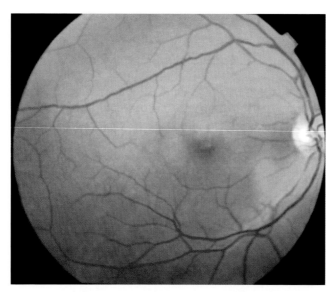

FIGURE 1.48: Parafoveal telangiectasia
A zone of retinal whitening above and temporal to the macula

Lately, a new terminology, Idiopathic Macular Telangiectasia (IMT) has been suggested along with a new classification. Accordingly, the patients have been categorized into two types: *type-1 (Figures 1.47A and B)* or aneurysmal telangiectasia; and *type-2* or perifoveal telangiectasia *(Figure 1.48)*.

Fundus fluorescein angiography. Type-1 cases show microaneurysmal and saccular dilatation of the temporal parafoveal capillaries *(Figure 1.47B)*. Fluorescein angiogram of case with Type-2 IMT shows dilated parafoveal capillaries with staining of the adjacent retina in late phases. Right-angled venules are better visualized *(Figures 1.49A to I)*.

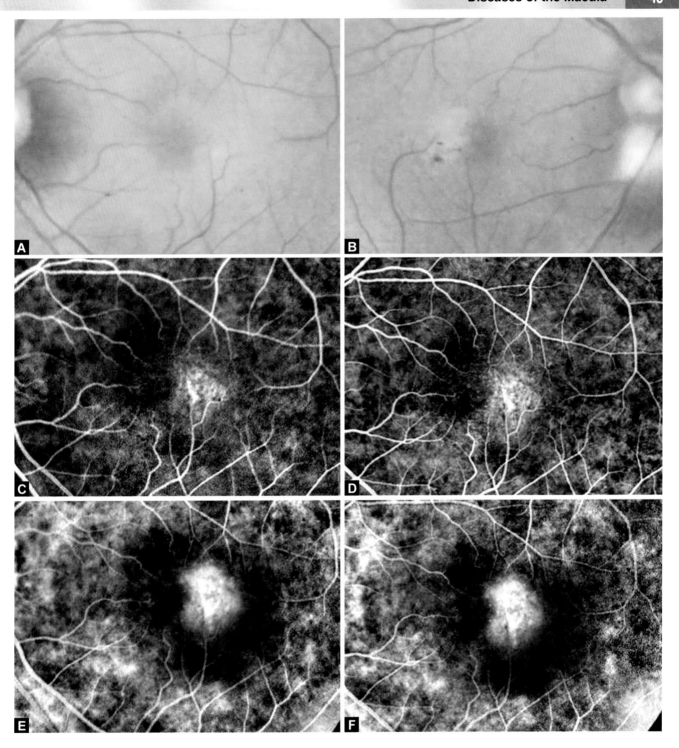

FIGURES 1.49A to F

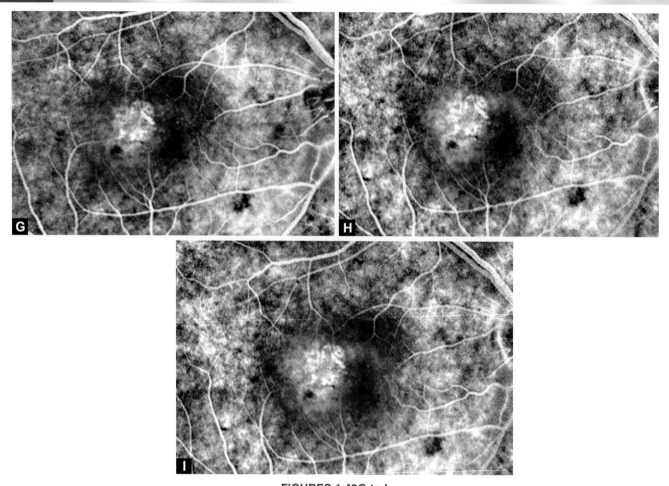

FIGURES 1.49G to I
FIGURES A to I: Parafoveal telangiectasia
Bilateral PFT, angiogram shows dilated parafoveal capillaries in the early phase with staining of the retina around the capillaries in late phases; right-angled veins are present

Treatment

Laser photocoagulation may benefit certain categories of the condition such as lesions localized to a small zone temporal to the fovea.

Intravitreal injection of Avastin has been advocated in the complicated cases of PFT. A randomized clinical trial is ongoing to study the efficacy of Lucentis in the treatment of the parafoveal telagiectatic lesions.

10. CHOROIDAL NEOVASCULAR MEMBRANE (OTHER THAN ARMD)

CNV may also be seen in conditions other than ARMD. Some of these conditions include degenerative myopia *(Figure 1.50)*, traumatic choroidal ruptures *(Figures 1.51A to I)*, presumed ocular histoplasmosis syndrome (POHS), and angioid streaks. Frequently, it may be idiopathic in nature *(Figures 1.52A to D)*. The membrane may be located in the subfoveal, juxtafoveal, parafoveal region, or juxtapapillary region *(Figures 1.53A to F)*.

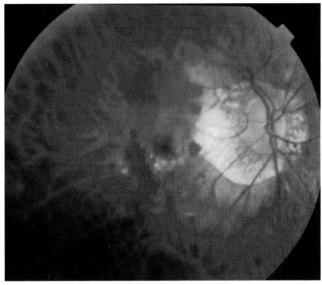

FIGURE 1.50: Choroidal neovascularization other than age-related macular degeneration
CNV in myopia

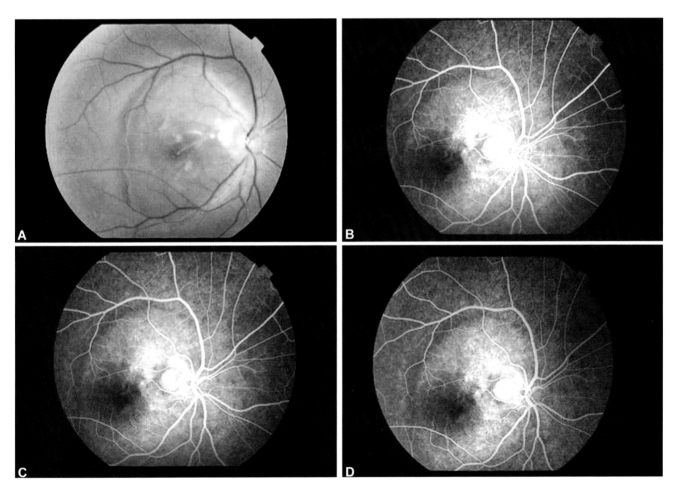

FIGURES 1.51A to D

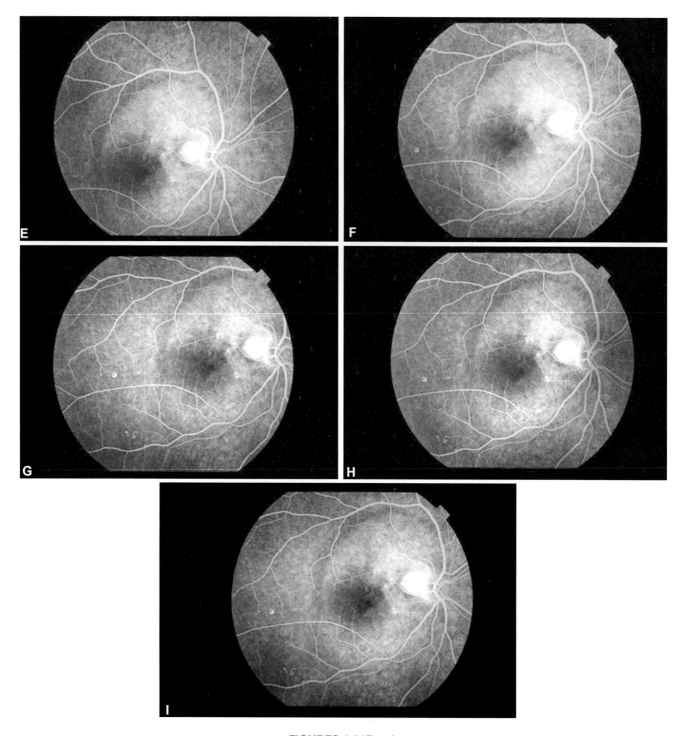

FIGURES 1.51E to I
FIGURES A to I: Choroidal neovascularization other than age-related macular degeneration
CNV in healed choroidal rupture

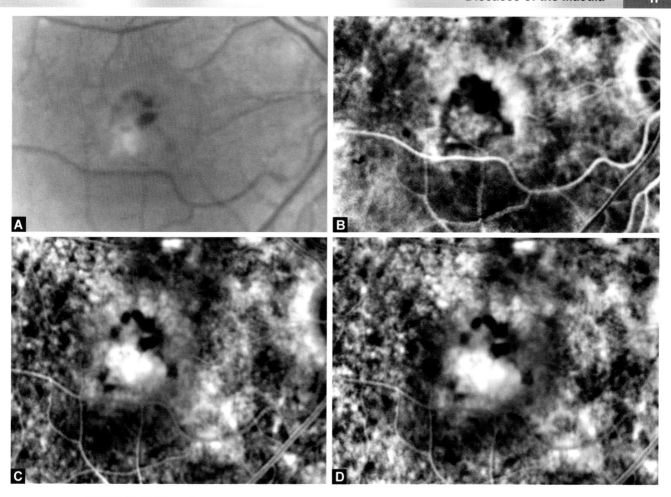

FIGURES 1.52A to D: Choroidal neovascularization other than age-related macular degeneration
Idiopathic CNV

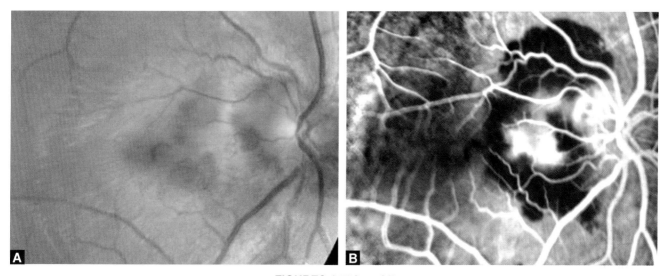

FIGURES 1.53A and B

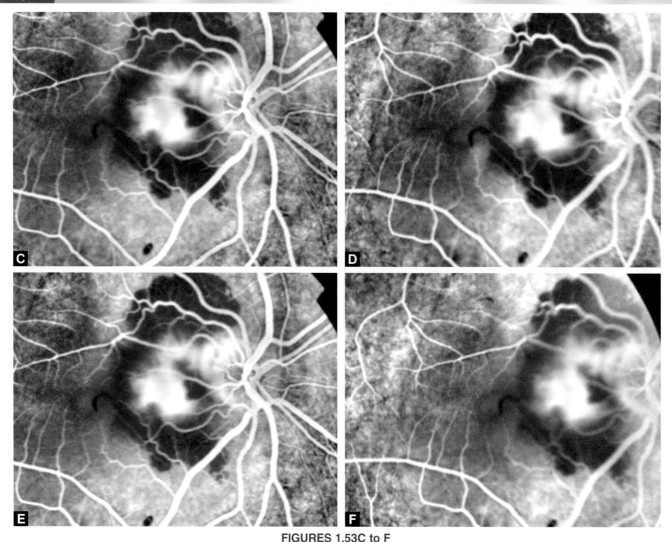

FIGURES 1.53C to F
FIGURES A to F: Choroidal neovascularization other than age-related macular degeneration
Idiopathic, juxtapapillary CNV

11. CHOROIDAL FOLDS

Choroidal folds are occasionally seen at the posterior pole that may be in the form of coarse folds *(Figure 1.54)*, or fine wrinkles. The folds may be idiopathic in nature, or associated with a number of conditions such as orbital tumors (particularly glioma or meningioma of optic nerve), thyroid eye disease, posterior scleritis, Vogt-Koyanagi-Harada disease, and papilledema. In the case of papilledema, choroidal folds tend to persist even after the disk swelling has disappeared. Final visual acuity is affected in most eyes.

Idiopathic syndrome of aquired hyperopia and choroidal folds has been described. Some of these cases were associated with intracranial hypertension with or without papilledema. Orbital imaging revealed flattening of the posterior pole of the globe, and distension of the perioptic subarachnoid space.

12. CHOROIDAL RUPTURE

Choroidal ruptures are the breaks in the chorid, Bruch's membrane, and the retinal pigment epithelium (RPE) that result from a direct or indirect trauma to the eye. Ruptures secondary to direct trauma tend to be placed

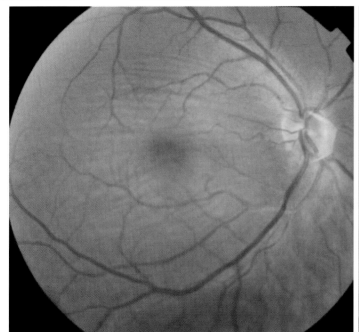 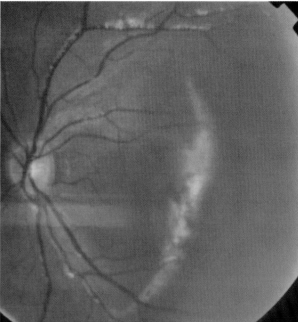

FIGURE 1.54: Choroidal folds
Horizontally placed choroidal folds resulting from space-occupying lesion of orbit

FIGURE 1.55: Choroidal rupture
White crescentric lesion

peripherally, parallel to the ora serrata, while those from direct trauma are located posteriorly. Choroidal ruptures resulting from indirect trauma are crescent shaped, and are placed parallel to the optic disk. Choroidal ruptures from indirect trauma are 5 times more common than those resulting from direct trauma. Occasionally, the ruptures may be multiple in the traumatized eye.

The impact of blunt trauma compresses the eyeball acutely followed by a sudden hyperextension. Because of its tensile strength, sclera escapes along with retina because of its elasticity. Bruch's membrane breaks, as it does not possess the required degree of tensile strength, or the elasticity. Concurrently, the choriocapillaries get damaged causing subretinal, or sub-RPE hemorrhage. The deep choroidal vessels usually escape. In the acute phase, the ruptures may be masked by the hemorrhage and retinal edema. In the healed stage, the choroidal rupture appears as a white, crescentric scar placed concentric to the disk, and showing variable amount of pigmentation *(Figure 1.55)*.

During the healing phase, choroidal vascularization (CNV) may occur *(see Figures 1.51A to I)*. In most cases, these vessels undergo spontaneous involution. However, in 15-30% cases, CNV recurs, usually within the first year of trauma, and leads to hemorrhage or serous detachment of macula resulting in significant visual loss. If the rupture does not involve the fovea, good vision is expected.

Fundus fluorescein angiography (FFA) is of help to diagnose the development of CNV. Indocyanin green angiography (ICGA) is the procedure of choice if hemorrhage blocks or hides the CNV on FFA.

Treatment

Conservative treatment is required in most cases, during the acute phase of the rupture. Early CNV resolves spontaneously in most cases, but recurs in 15-30% cases. Extrafoveal CNV may be treated with direct conventional laser. The results of photodynamic therapy (PDT) are reported to be inconsistent. Pars plana vitrectomy with membrane extraction has been suggested for treating the subfoveal CNV.

13. MACULAR HEMORRAHAGE

It is not a disease entity *per se*, but the result of a host of ocular or systemic disease. Usually of sudden occurrence, it accompanies a profound loss of central vision. The ultimate visual prognosis depends on the intensity of the hemorrhage and the underlying cause. Generally, it is located in the retinal tissue itself, in the choroids *(see Figures 1.24A and B)*, or may be preretinal (subhyaloid—*Figures 1.56A and B).*

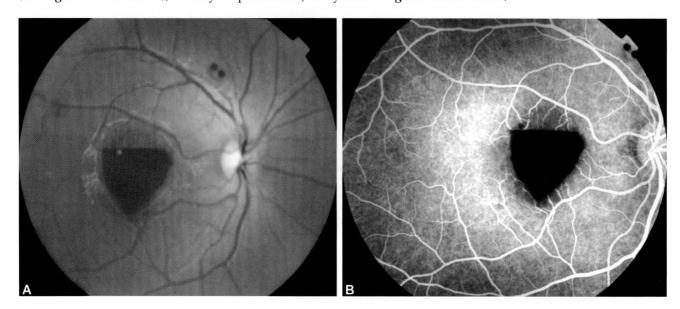

FIGURES 1.56A and B: Subhyaloid hemorrhage
A. Subhyaloid hemorrhage at the macula with a level or flat top
B. Masked fluorescence in the angiogram

Treatment

Treatment consists of the management of the causative disease.

14. COMMOTIO RETINAE (BERLIN'S EDEMA)

It is the result of concussion of the neuroretina following a blunt trauma to the eyeball. It manifests as whitening of the retina, mostly on the temporal side *(Figures 1.57A and B).* The cloudy appearance manifests as the result of the disruption of the outer segments of photoreceptors. Extracellular edema has not been demonstrated in the animal models. The macula frequently gives rise to 'cherry red' spot appearance. A mild degree of retinal opacification may disappear without any sequel or any significant visual damage. Severe forms may be followed by degenerative changes at the macula, or the formation of a macular hole.

Treatment

There is no treatment for commotion retinae. Various kinds of collateral damage are managed on its merits. Development of cystoid macular edema is a serious complication with variable response to injected steroidal depots.

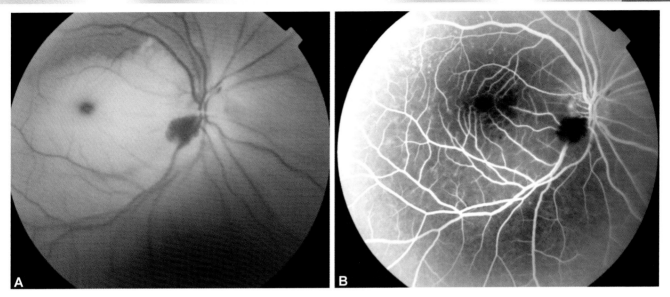

FIGURES 1.57A and B: Commotio retinae
A. Whitening of the retina at the posterior pole with cherry-red spot
B. Normally filling retinal vessels in the angiogram; hypofluorescence at the optic disk is due to hemorrhage

15. EPIMACULAR MEMBRANE (EMM)

The epimacular membranes are avascular, fibrocellular membranes that proliferate on the inner surface of the central retina. The membranes have contractile properties and are responsible for varying degrees of visual disturbance, because of their wrinkling effect on the underlying retina. The effect on vision depends upon the severity of retinal distortion, the location, and other secondary effects on the retina. The membranes are known by different names, such as cellophane maculopathy, surface wrinkling maculopathy, silkscreen maculopathy, preretinal macular fibrosis, and macular pucker.

EMMs are associated with a variety of ocular conditions, such as posterior vitreous detachment (PVD), retinal breaks, retinal detachment, retinal vascular occlusive disease, diabetic retinopathy, ocular inflammations, and vitreous hemorrhage. EMM may also result from certain retinal procedures such as surgery for retinal detachment, photocoagulation, and retinal cryopexy. However, large proportions of membranes have no obvious association with such conditions and, therefore, are classified as idiopathic epimacular membranes (IEMM). Post-retinal detachment membranes along with IEMMs constitute the largest group of EMMs.

Vitrectomy specimens show that the type of cells, responsible for the proliferation of the membrane, include glial cells, retinal pigment epithelial cells, fibroblasts, and collagen cells. The proportion of various cells varies according to the etiology of the membrane formation. Membranes associated with retinal breaks, retinal detachment, or retinal cryopexy are composed of mainly the dispersed retinal pigment epithelial cells, while cells of glial origin predominate in idiopathic membranes.

In the initial stages, the membrane may not cause any symptoms. As the membrane progresses, distortion and blurring of vision are the common complaints. In advanced cases, metamorphopsia, micropsia, and Amsler's grid anomalies are present. There is a marked reduction of vision in postretinal detachment membranes.

Fundus appearance of the membranes may vary according to the degree of severity. Accordingly, the membranes are categorized as:

Grade 0 membrane: This is a translucent membrane, not associated with retinal distortion. This condition is referred to as cellophane maculopathy.

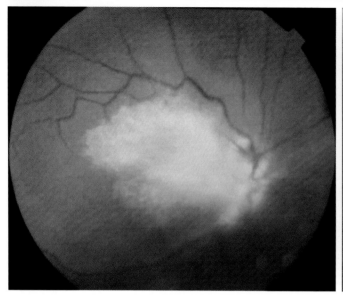

FIGURE 1.58: Epiretinal membrane
Translucent membrane over the macula and surrounding retina

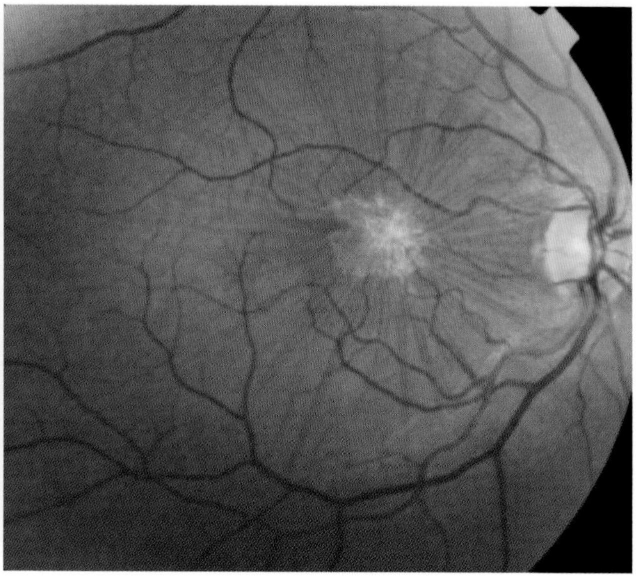

FIGURE 1.59: Epiretinal membrane
Opaque, thick epiretinal membrane at the macula; gross wrinkling of the retina around the membrane

Grade 1 membrane: The membrane causes an irregular wrinkling of the inner surface of the retina. Fine, superficial radiating folds extend outward from the margins of the membrane. Wrinkling of the retina may be sufficient to cause tortuosity of the paramacular vessels, pulling them toward macula *(Figure 1.58)*.

Grade 2 membrane: The membrane, especially after retinal detachment, has an opaque, thick appearance. There is full-thickness wrinkling of the macula along with retinal edema, small hemorrhages, and cotton wool spots. This condition is designated as macular pucker *(Figure 1.59)*.

Treatment

There is no medical treatment for epiretinal membranes.

Surgical treatment consists of pars plana vitrectomy followed by epiretinal membrane peeling. The procedure of peeling consists, essentially, of identifying the outer edge of the membrane and creating a dissection plane, with the use of a blunt pick or bent needle. Once the edge of the membrane is visualized, it is gently lifted off the retinal surface, in tangential manner, with the use of the pick or fine forceps. Thick membranes are peeled inside-out by slitting the membrane in the middle and, thus, creating an edge for the subsequent maneuver, in a circular fashion, not unlike the technique of continuous circular capsulorhexis. There is an opinion that virectomy should be avoided in the surgery of membrane peeling because of a high incidence of rapidly developing cataracts in the postvitrectomy eyes. However, vitrectomy has the advantage of preventing vitreous contraction, and removes all traction on the macula.

Surgical removal of the epiretinal membranes generally results in both improvement of vision and the biomicroscopic appearance of the macula. Sometimes, however, metamorphopsia may persist despite improvement in visual acuity. This is seen mostly in the cases in which there is an incomplete peeling of the membrane. On the contrary, metamorphopsia may improve but with a poor visual return. This is seen in the eyes with a longstanding macular edema before the surgery.

Chapter 2

Retinal Vascular Diseases

1. ARTERIAL OCCLUSIONS

Arterial occlusions occur more commonly in elderly people as the result of embolic phenomenon and thrombosis (atherosclerosis). Peri-arteritis as seen in certain collagen diseases such as systemic lupus erythematosis, and peri-arteritis nodosa may also cause branch arterial occlusions. Occasionally, it may be seen in certain blood dyscrasias (e.g. sickle cell anemia), and rarely, in migraine. Rarely, it may result from orbital hemorrhage or cellulitis. The resultant clinical picture depends upon the site and extent of occlusion.

Classification

Central Retinal Artery Occlusion (CRAO)

Central retinal artery occlusion (CRAO) presents with a profound unilateral loss of vision, of sudden onset. It is ophthalmic emergency, and delay in treatment may result in permanent loss of vision. Some amount of central vision may be spared in the eyes with cilioretinal artery. Bilateral involvement is rare and is suggestive of embolic origin or temporal arteritis. Atherosclerosis is the leading cause of CRAO in patients aged 40-60 years, while embolus from the heart is the most common cause in patients below 40 years, and coagulopathy from sickle cell anemia in patients below 30 years. Of all the cases of retinal arterial occlusions, CRAO occurs in 57%.

On examination, Marcus-Gunn pupil (relative afferent papillary conduction defect) is present. The retina has a white appearance because of cloudy swelling of the retina caused by an intracellular edema. The fovea appears orange-red ('cherry red spot') because of the absence of inner retinal layers in this zone, with the normally perfused choroid in the background *(Figures 2.1A and B)*. There is marked narrowing of the arteries as well as the veins, and segmentation of the blood column in the vessels may be present *(Figures 2.2A and B)*. If the occlusion persists, the whitening of retina and the 'cherry red' spot disappear in a few weeks' time. The attenuation of the vessels, however, persists. The optic disk becomes white and atrophic *(Figure 2.3)*. It is uncommon to see the development of rubeosis of the iris and secondary glaucoma.

Fundus Fluorescein Angiography

In acute cases, hypofluorescence is present in the central retina caused by the cloudy swelling of the retina in the area. Arterial phase is extremely delayed and there is marked delay in the arteriovenous transit time. Arterial blood column may be broken causing cattle-truck appearance *(Figure 2.2B)*.

Branch Retinal Artery Occlusion (BRAO)

Branch retinal artery occlusion (BRAO) is generally caused by the emboli of various origins *(Figures 2.4A to I)*. The most common site of obstruction is the arteriovenous junction. Although small, peripheral 'micro-infarcts' may be asymptomatic, the most common presentation is in the form of the patient's complaint of altitudinal field defect corresponding to the region of retinal infarction. A cloudy swelling of the retina is present in the

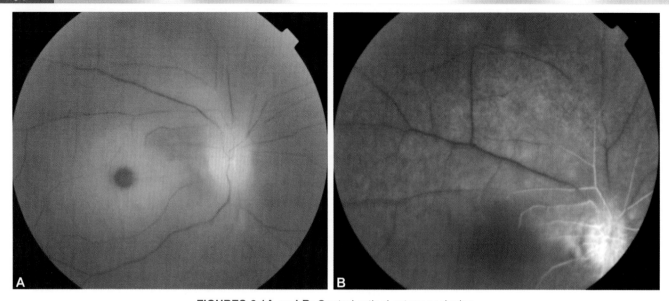

FIGURES 2.1A and B: Central retinal artery occlusion
A. Thread-like arteries, narrow veins, whitening of retina at the posterior pole, and cherry red spot at the macula
B. Delayed and incomplete filling of narrow arteries; veins are still devoid of dye

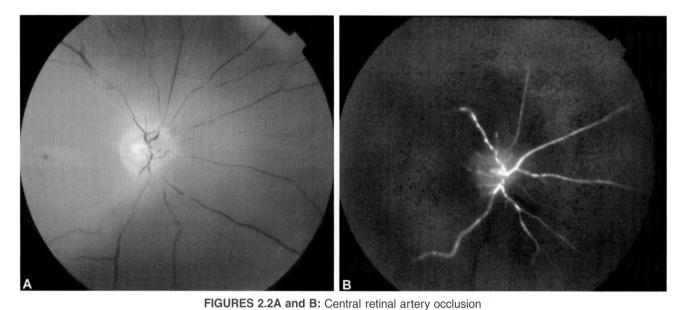

FIGURES 2.2A and B: Central retinal artery occlusion
A. Segmentation of blood column in narrowed arteries and veins; fading posterior pole whitening, and cherry red spot
B. Angiogram shows segmentation of blood in arteries; filling of arteries with fluorescein is delayed and incomplete

area supplied by the occluded vessel. The whitening of the retina disappears in a few weeks' time, but the involved retina becomes atrophic leaving behind a permanent field defect. BRAO accounts for 38% of all retinal arterial occlusions.

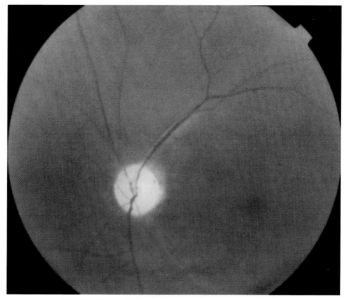

FIGURE 2.3: Central retinal artery occlusion
Narrow retinal vessels, especially the arteries with waxy pale optic disk
(consecutive optic atrophy) six months after the episode of arterial occlusion

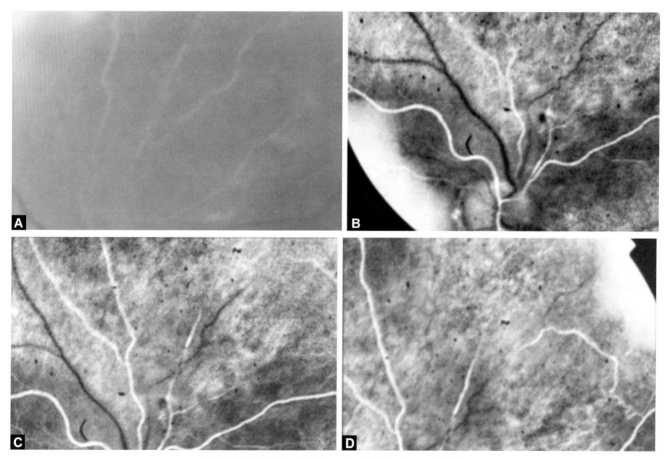

FIGURES 2.4A to D: Branch retinal artery occlusion
Clinical photograph shows thin whitened branches in the upper nasal arterial tree; angiogram shows delayed and incomplete filling of dye in thread-like branches, intraretinal microvascular abnormalities (IRMA) and areas of NCP are visible

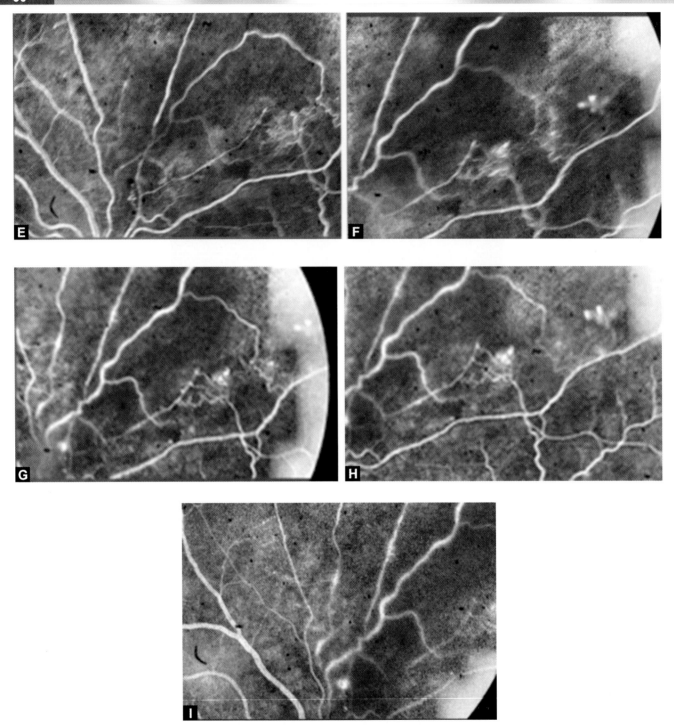

FIGURES 2.4E to I: Branch retinal artery occlusion
Clinical photograph shows thin whitened branches in the upper nasal arterial tree; angiogram shows delayed and incomplete filling of dye in thread-like branches, intraretinal microvascular abnormalities (IRMA) and areas of NCP are visible

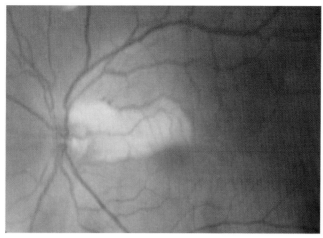

FIGURE 2.5: Cilioretinal artery occlusion
Whitening of the retinal zone perfused by the occluded cilioretinal artery

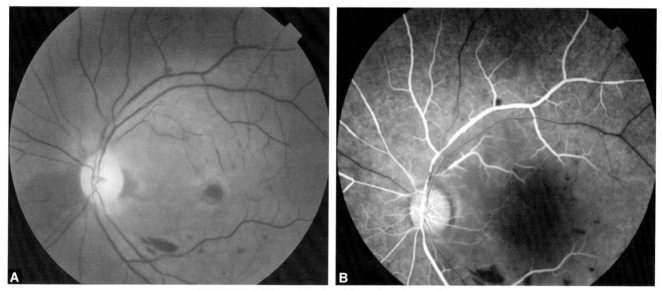

FIGURES 2.6A and B: Combined CRAO and CRVO
A. Narrow retinal arteries, especially on the optic disk; fading posterior pole whitening and cherry red spot; retinal hemorrhages
B. Angiogram shows obstruction in the arteries at and around the optic disk; delayed filling of the arterial tree; absence of small arterioles; delayed and incomplete filling of veins; ischemic macula

Cilioretinal Artery Occlusion

The cilioretinal artery, derived from the posterior ciliary arterial system, is present in many eyes. A single or 2-3 arteries may be present. It perfuses the retina at the posterior pole. The occlusion of this vessel causes a variable amount of the loss of central vision, while the peripheral vision is normal. The resultant retinal whitening is confined to the area of its perfusion *(Figure 2.5).* The prevalence of cilioretinal artery occlusion is 5% of all arterial occlusions.

Combined CRAO-CRVO Occlusion

On rare occasions, the common risk factors for the venous and arterial occlusions are responsible for causing the occlusive phenomenon simultaneously in the retinal vein as well as the artery *(Figures 2.6A and B).*

Treatment

The main aim of the treatment is to re-establish or improve circulation in the closed vessel. Although the retinal tissue cannot survive the loss of blood supply beyond a few hours, the treatment may be undertaken within forty-eight hours, or even later, because the occlusion of arteries seldom causes a complete closure. No randomized clinical trials have been made to compare the results of a particular modality of treatment with any other form of treatment that are recommended in anecdotal reports and case series.

Ocular massage is performed by applying pressure on the eyeball with fingers for 5-15 seconds and then releasing the pressure. The procedure is to be repeated several times, for 5-10 minutes. Sudden drop in intra-ocular pressure on releasing the pressure, increases the volume of flow, and may dislodge the embolus to a point further down the arterial circulation.

Anterior chamber paracentesis has been advocated if the ocular massage fails to succeed, or even as the primary procedure, if the visual loss has been present for less than 24 hours.

Carbogen therapy (5% carbon dioxide, 95% oxygen) is aimed at dilatation of the arteries caused by carbon dioxide, and oxygen supplementation to the ischemic tissues.

Thrombolytic drugs may be useful if the treatment is initiated within 4-6 hours of visual loss.

Hyperbaric oxygen is believed to be beneficial if administered within 2-12 hours of the episode. A controlled study has reported the benefit seen in the treated group.

Drugs used for treating the acute angle closure glaucoma such as acetazolamide, dorzolamide, and intravenous mannitol, have been recommended to achieve reduction of intraocular pressure.

The patient may be asked to breathe into a paper bag to increase blood carbon dioxide level that may induce vasodilatation. Overall, the result of any treatment is mostly disappointing.

2. VENOUS OCCLUSIONS

Venous occlusions are seen much more frequently than the arterial occlusions. Thrombus formation is the most common underlying factor that is predisposed by a systemic hypertension, in aged persons. In the young, however, inflammatory phenomenon is the dominant factor. A central vein occlusion (CRVO) results if the obstruction to venous flow is located at the level of lamina cribrosa. Central retinal artery and vein share a common adventitial sheath as they pass through a narrow opening in the lamina cribrosa, thus providing little space for displacement and producing a compartment syndrome. The vein gets compressed by the abnormally thickened arterial wall (as in arteriosclerosis), causing hemodynamic changes, endothelial damage and thrombus formation. It has been reported that the fellow eye may develop retinal vein occlusion in about 7% cases within 2 years, the incidence increasing with time.

Branch retinal vein occlusions (BRVO) signify the involvement of one of the major (temporal or nasal) veins *(Figure 2.7)*, or their tributaries—*tributary vein occlusion (Figures 2.8A and B)*, which include the macular branch—*macular branch occlusion (Figures 2.9A and B).* The obstruction of flow in the main upper or lower branch causes a *hemispherical vein occlusion (Figure 2.10).*

Central Retinal Vein Occlusion (CRVO)

Based on the clinical picture and the prognostic considerations, the central retinal vein occlusion is classified as *non-ischemic* and *ischemic* types. Such a distinction is made on the basis of visual acuity at presentation, presence or absence of relative afferent papillary defect (RAPD), extent of retinal hemorrhage and cotton-wool spots, extent of retinal non-perfusion on fluorescein angiography, and electroretinographic changes.

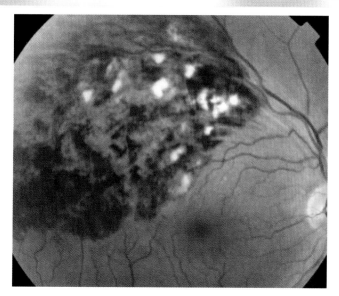

FIGURE 2.7: Branch retinal vein occlusion
Occlusion of the superotemporal branch of central retinal vein with densely placed retinal hemorrhages in the zone of its drainage; several cotton-wool spots are seen; macula is spared

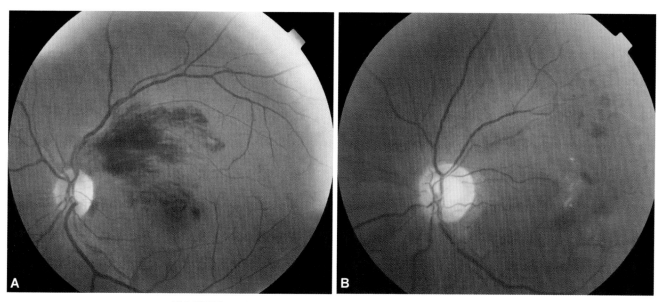

FIGURES 2.8A and B: Tributary branch retinal vein occlusion
A. Occlusion of a centrally placed tributary of superior temporal vein
B. Occlusion of a peripheral tributary

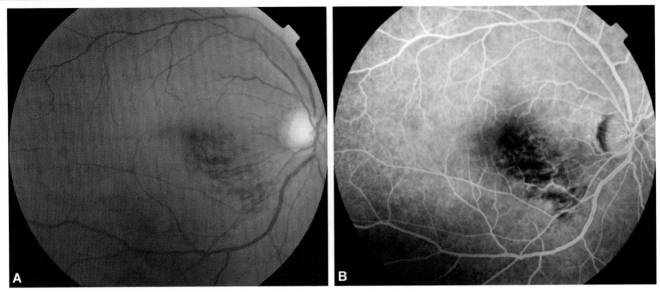

FIGURES 2.9A and B: Macular branch retinal vein occlusion
A. Occlusion of a small tributary of inferotemporal vein draining the macular area
B. Angiogram shows the site of occlusion at the arteriovenous crossing with
hypofluorescence caused by the retinal hemorrhages

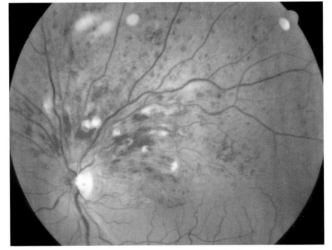

FIGURE 2.10: Hemispherical central retinal vein occlusion
Occlusion of the upper division of central retinal vein that includes both the upper temporal and upper nasal branches

Non-ischemic CRVO

Non-ischemic CRVO is the most common type of occlusion, seen in nearly three quarters of all cases, and represents occlusion of the central retinal vein without significant retinal ischemia.

It presents with a mild-to-moderate loss of vision. Slight relative afferent pupillary defect may be detected. Fundus picture shows a few, to many retinal hemorrhages distributed throughout the retina *(Figures 2.11A and B).* Cotton-wool patches are usually absent. There may be mild-to-moderate hyperemia and swelling of

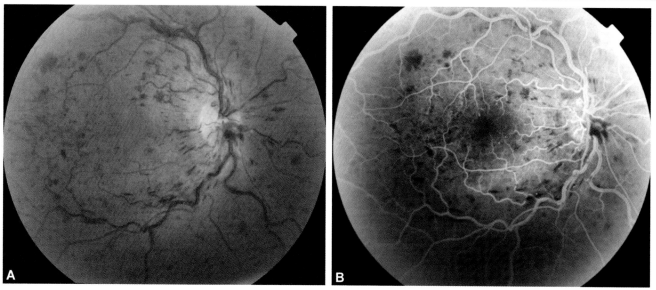

FIGURES 2.11A and B: Non-ischemic central retinal vein occlusion
A. Engorged central retinal vein, several retinal hemorrhages, no cotton-wool spots, no swelling of the optic disk
B. Angiogram shows spots of hypofluorescence corresponding to retinal hemorrhages,
no leakage of dye from the optic disk, no areas of NCP, well-perfused macula

the optic disk. Macular edema, if present, is of mild intensity. Visual prognosis is relatively good, unless chronic cystoid macular edema results in a permanent damage to the central foveal area. Complete recovery with good visual acuity occurs in nearly 10% cases and 50% eyes have a visual acuity of 6/60 or less. About 1/3 cases convert to ischemic CRVO in 3 years; 15% within 4 months. A regular follow-up examination is, therefore, essential. Fluorescein angiographic examination is made every 4 months to assess the status of macular edema and retinal non-perfusion. Simultaneously, a gonioscopic examination is to be carried out to detect the development of new vessels.

Fundus fluorescein angiography reveals multiple areas of blocked fluorescence because of the retinal hemorrhages. Veins appear tortuous and engorged.

A relatively uncommon condition of *papillophlebitis* is seen in young adults without any systemic disease. It is essentially a CRVO in young, healthy patient, believed to be the result of inflammation of retinal or papillary vessels and also referred as *optic disk vasculitis*. The clinical picture and its course are typically benign but, some eyes may develop persistent macular edema and neovascular complications as seen in ischemic CRVO. The ultimate prognosis is good in a large majority of cases. No effective treatment is known. The response to systemic corticosteroids is unequivocal.

Partial occlusion of the central retinal vein is seen occasionally. It manifests as engorged veins with a few retinal hemorrhages *(Figure 2.12A)*. The condition may remain asymptomatic, or cause mild visual disturbance, unless there is development of macular edema *(Figure 2.12B)* that causes a profound loss of vision. The condition is also referred as venous stasis retinopathy.

Treatment

Treatment of non-ischemic venous occlusions is indicated in the situation where cystoid macular edema or a later development of new vessels (NVE or NVD) is detected. Cystoid macular edema is often resistant to treatment. Modalities of treatment for these complications are described with the treatment of ischemic CRVO.

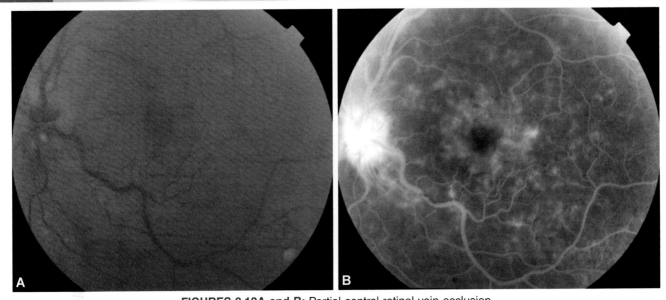

FIGURES 2.12A and B: Partial central retinal vein occlusion
A. Chronic stasis in the central retinal vein causing engorgement of veins, a few hemorrhages, thickening of central retina
B. Angiogram shows cystoid macular edema, several spots of hyperfluorescence due to leakage of dye causing diffuse edema at the posterior pole

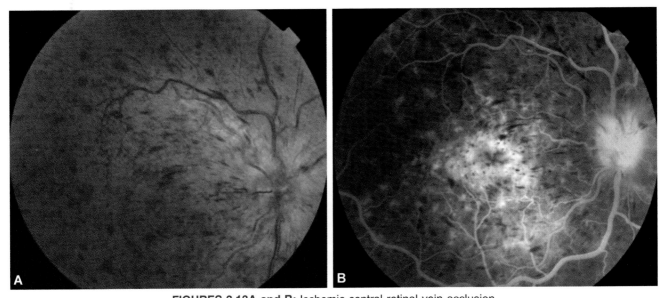

FIGURES 2.13A and B: Ischemic central retinal vein occlusion
A. Extensive retinal hemorrhages causing 'battle-field' appearance of retina, swelling of optic disk, macular edema
B. Angiogram shows hyperfluorescent optic disk, several spots of hyperfluorescence in the central retina suggestive of edema of the posterior pole with cystoid pattern at the macula

Ischemic CRVO

Ischemic CRVO is less common than the non-ischemic variety, and presents with a profound, unilateral loss of vision of sudden origin. The visual acuity is reduced to 6/60 or less. There is a marked degree of relative afferent papillary defect. Fundus appearance shows a marked engorgement and tortuosity of the veins along with extensive retinal hemorrhages involving both the peripheral and the central retina *(Figure 2.13A and B)*. Cotton-wool spots are usually present, and the optic disk shows a marked hyperemia and swelling. A significant amount of macular edema is seen in most cases. More than 90% patients will have visual acuity of 6/60 or worse. About 60% develop ocular neovascularization with associated complications.

Fluorescein angiography may not be very informative in the acute phase of the occlusion because of the extensive hemorrhages that mask the visualization of angiographic features. However, it shows all the features as described in the case of non-ischemic CRVO. In addition, there is a markedly delayed filling of the veins. Extensive areas of capillary non-perfusion (CNP) may be visualized, which may extend to the macular area.

Fundus fluorescein angiography (FFA) is a very useful investigation for the evaluation of retinal capillary perfusion *(Figure 2.14)*, posterior segment neovascularization *(Figure 2.15)*, and macular edema *(Figure 2.16)*.

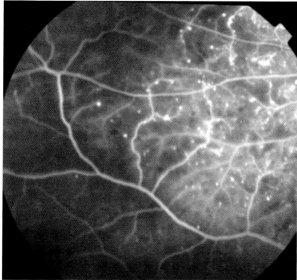

FIGURE 2.14: Ischemic central retinal vein occlusion Angiogram showing extensive areas of NCP in the peripheral retina

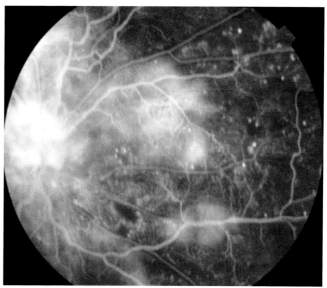

FIGURE 2.15: Ischemic central retinal vein occlusion Angiogram of a case of ischemic CRVO shows extensive areas of hyperfluorescence at the optic disk and surrounding retina because of leakage of fluorescein from NVD and NVE

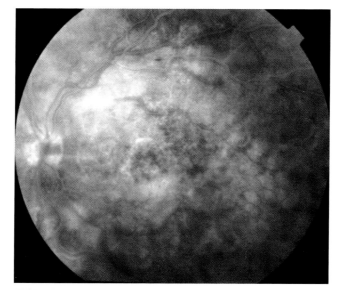

FIGURE 2.16: Macular edema in central retinal vein occlusion Angiogram of an old case of CRVO showing diffuse hyperfluorescence at the posterior pole—persistent macular edema

In recent cases, however, the reliability of the findings is hampered by the large number of retinal hemorrhages. FFA provides one of the important criteria employed to classify cases of CRVO into the ischemic or non-ischemic category. A non-perfused area of 10 disk diameters or more is suggestive of ischemic CRVO.

Optical coherence tomography (OCT) is helpful to diagnose macular edema despite the presence of widespread and dense retinal hemorrhages. Its ability to make quantitative assessment of the swelling provides a valuable guide in monitoring the response to treatment.

Electroretinography (ERG). Amplitude of b wave is decreased, relative to the a wave. Some studies indicate that the b-to-a wave ratio of less than 1 is indicative of ischemic CRVO.

Treatment Earlier attempts to treat cases of CRVO with anticoagulants, fibrinolytic agents, etc. did not succeed. The current treatment modalities available include intraocular or periocular administration of corticosteroids, VEGF inhibitors, laser coagulation, and pars plana vitrectomy along with some newer surgical procedures.

Intravitreal injection of triamcinolone acetonide has been observed to be an effective procedure in the treatment of macular edema. Doses of 4-25 mg have been used. Multiple treatments are usually required. There are reports suggesting that peribulbar, subTenon deposition of the drug may be equally effective. A bio-degradable, long-acting intravitreal implant of dexamethasone is under investigation. Preliminary reports are encouraging. Complications of corticosteroid therapy include cataract formation, rise in IOP, infective or non-infective endophthalmitis, and retinal detachment.

The role of VEGF inhibitors in the treatment of post-occlusion macular edema provides an exciting and promising possibility. Intravitreal injection of VEGF inhibitors like Avastin has been used with good results in eyes with recurrent or persistent macular edema. The treatment may have to be repeated.

Laser treatment consists of grid pattern photocoagulation, provided macular ischemia has been excluded on fluorescein angiography. Although grid laser may succeed in relieving edema at the macula, it does not improve the visual acuity. Panretinal photocoagulation (PRP) is performed in the event of the development of neovascularization in the retina, the optic disk or on the iris. According to the guidelines provided by the central venous occlusion study (CVOS):

- Prophylactic PRP, performed in eyes with 10 or more disk areas of retinal capillary nonperfusion, does not prevent neovascularization and recommends waiting for the development of early neovascularization and then applying PRP.
- Argon laser is usually used. Laser spots of about 500 micron, 0.1-0.2 second duration with sufficient power to give medium white burns, are placed around the posterior pole extending anteriorly to equator. A total of 1,200 to 2,500 spots are placed, one burn apart.
- If ocular media is hazy for laser coagulation, cryoablation of the peripheral fundus is performed by applying 16-32 trans-scleral cryospots from ora serrata posteriorly.
- At present, results of the study do not support a recommendation for grid coagulation for macular edema.

Pars plana vitrectomy is seldom required to treat eyes with CRVO. Pars plana vitrectomy with or without peeling of the internal limiting membrane (ILM) has been reported to reduce macular edema, and improve visual acuity in cases of CRVO. According to one theory, the procedure acts by relieving traction on the macula. An other hypothesis suggests that removal of vitreous gets rid of the cytokines and VEGF associated with a venous obstructive event.

Chorioretinal venous anastomosis has been attempted to bypass the site of venous obstruction in the optic nerve. The procedure consists of puncturing the retinal veins, either by using laser or by surgery, through the RPE and Bruch's membrane into the choroid. The anastomosis so produced tends to reduce macular edema. The reported success rate is low and the procedure is not free of possible serious complications. The indication and the timing have not been clearly indicated.

Radial optic neurotomy is a new technique in which a microvitreal blade is used during pars plana vitrectomy, to relax the scleral ring around the optic nerve. It is suggested that it decompresses the closed compartment and leads to improved venous outflow and reduction in the amount of macular edema. The results have been inconsistent and there is no consensus for the use of this technique.

Branch Retinal Vein Occlusion

Arterial compression of the vein at the arteriovenous crossing, is believed to be the underlying cause of BRVO. Turbulence of flow in the vein caused by the compression combines with the pre-existing vascular endothelial damage from the different conditions (systemic hypertension, diabetes, and atherosclerosis, etc.) to facilitate intravascular thrombus formation. Therefore, BRVO almost always occurs at the site of an arteriovenous crossing *(Figure 2.17)*. The occlusion is most common in the superotemporal branch probably because of the greater number of arteriovenous crossings in this quadrant. Occlusions of the nasal branches are minimally symptomatic.

Occasionally, inflammations like sarcoidosis, serpiginous choroiditis, and rarely, thrombophilic conditions like deficiency of protein S or C, and antithrombin factor III may be the underlying factors causing BRVO.

The condition affects both the sexes equally, most commonly in the fifth or sixth decade. No racial predilection has been observed. Risk factors include systemic hypertension, diabetes, oral contraceptive intake in women, and pre-existing open angle glaucoma. A moderate amount of alcohol intake reduces the risk of BRVO.

The patient complains of visual symptoms varying from a slight blur to a considerable drop in central vision. The involved vessel appears engorged and tortuous along with deep and superficial retinal hemorrhages in the area of its drainage *(Figure 2.18)*. Some amount of retinal edema and cotton-wool spots are seen. In the occlusions of temporal vessels macular area is commonly involved in the form of hemorrhages, edema, or both, causing a reduced visual acuity. Later, in its course, in around 6 months, there is development of venous collaterals *(Figure 2.19A and B)* such that the ischemia is adequately compensated and the visual acuity improves to 6/12 or more. In the eyes where the collaterals fail to compensate for ischemia, new vessels develop in the

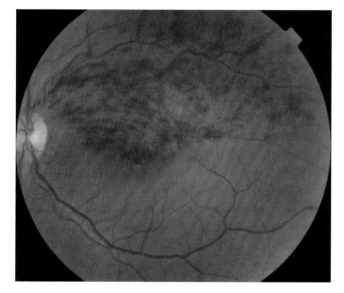

FIGURE 2.17: Branch retinal vein occlusion
Occlusion of the superotemporal vein at
the arteriovenous crossing

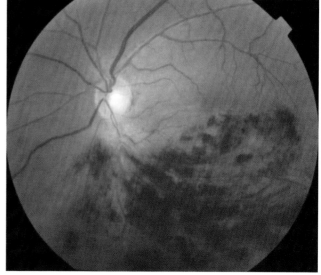

FIGURE 2.18: Branch retinal vein occlusion
Occlusion of inferotemporal vein with dense hemorrhages in
the zone of its drainage, macular edema is present

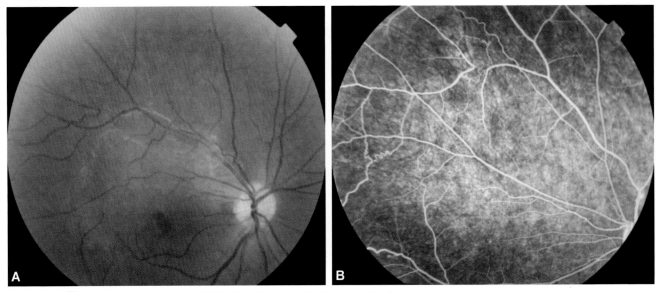

FIGURES 2.19A and B: Branch retinal vein occlusion
A. Old BRVO with developing venous collaterals (IRMA) as an attempt to compensate for retinal ischemia
B. Angiogram shows IRMA in the temporal retina along with areas of NCP in the superior retinal zone

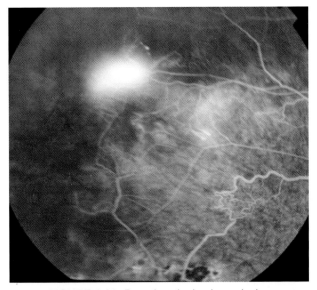

FIGURE 2.20: Branch retinal vein occlusion
Angiogram of an old BRVO showing large areas of NCP; hyperfluorescence caused by the leakage of dye from NVE at the border between the perfused and non-perfused areas of retina

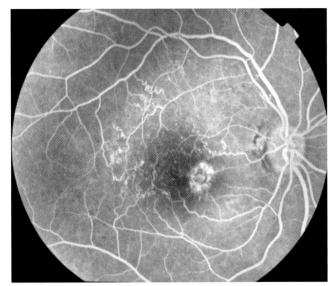

FIGURE 2.21: Branch retinal vein occlusion
Angiogram of an old BRVO shows perfused retina, venous collaterals; persisting macular edema resulted in poor visual acuity

retina *(Figure 2.20)* and occasionally, at the optic disk (NVD). A persistent macular edema *(Figure 2.21)* is the most common cause of reduced visual acuity in cases of BRVO.

Fluorescein angiography (Figure 2.22) shows masking of choroidal fluorescencec caused by the retinal hemorrhages. It is seen through all the phases. Filling of the occluded vein is delayed. Dilated capillaries and aneurysmal dilatations are visualized.

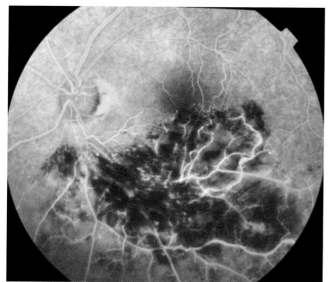

FIGURE 2.22: Branch retinal vein occlusion
Angiogram shows masked choroidal fluorescence because of
retinal hemorrhages; dilated capillaries with a few aneurysmal
dilatations

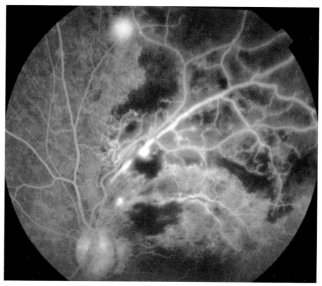

FIGURE 2.23: Branch retinal vein occlusion
Angiogram showing large areas (more than 5 DD)
of NCP—non-perfused BRVO

From the prognostic point of view, the retina is supposed to be adequately perfused if the extent of CNP is less than 5 disk diameters. In the eyes with CNP of 5 disk diameters or more, BRVO is considered as non-perfused *(Figure 2.23)*. Likewise, the macular edema is considered as perfused if an intact perifoveal network of capillaries is visualized in the arteriovenous phase followed by a leakage of the dye *(Figure 2.24)*; or *non-perfused* if the perifoveal capillaries are not visualized, and there is no subsequent leakage of the dye in the late phase *(Figures 2.25A and B)*. The state of non-perfusion of the perifoveal capillaries combined with capillary dilatation and leakage of dye is labeled as *mixed macular edema*. The recognition of the state of perfusion is important from the point of view of indication for the laser coagulation treatment in the cases, having a visual acuity of less than 6/12. Laser treatment is contraindicated in cases of non-perfused macular edema.

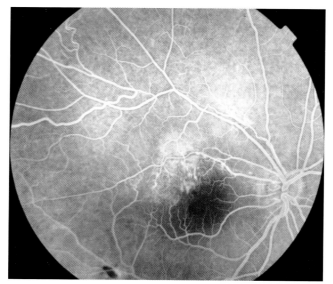

FIGURE 2.24: Branch retinal vein occlusion
Perfused macula with intact perifoveal capillary network; capillaries in the upper part of macula are
dilated with leakage of dye in this late phase angiogram

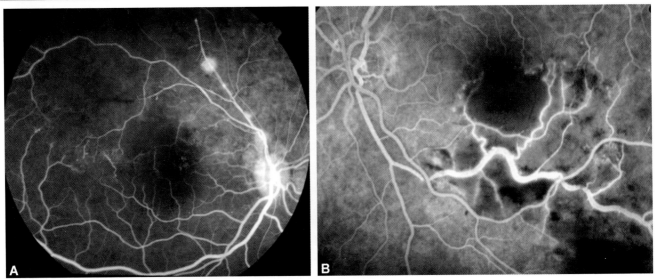

FIGURES 2.25A and B: Branch retinal vein occlusion
Non-perfused macula with loss of perifoveal capillary network

Treatment

Treatment is directed to manage the persistent macular edema, and NVE or NVD, if present. It is advised to wait for a spontaneous visual recovery for three months before steps are taken to treat macular edema. Fluorescein angiography is conducted to study the extent of edema, and to rule out macular ischemia. Optical coherence tomography (OCT) measures the retinal thickness in quantitative fashion, and is a useful adjunct in the follow up of patients.

The following guidelines have been suggested for laser treatment by the Branch Vein Occlusion Study (BVOS):
- Macular grid photocoagulation is mildly effective in the treatment of macular edema.
- It is recommended to wait for 3 months to see if the patient's vision improves spontaneously.
- If no visual improvement occurs and the hemorrhages have mostly cleared from the macular area, fluorescein angiogram is obtained. If it shows leakage in the macular area, macular grid photocoagulation is undertaken. After 3 years of follow up, 63% laser-treated eyes improved by 2 or more lines as compared with 36% of control eyes.

Laser treatment may be not warranted if the angiogram shows ischemia at the macula.

Macular edema is treated with the use of trimcinolone or VEGF inhibitors as recommended for the treatment of post-CRVO macular edema.

Macular branch vein thrombosis (Figures 2.9A and B) involves a small area in and around the macula. Visual acuity is usually compromised significantly. No ischemic changes, however, are caused in the retina. The prognosis is usually good depending largely on the status of the perifoveal capillaries. *Fluorescein angiography* shows areas of blocked fluorescence due to hemorrhages, delayed filling of the involved vein, and leakage of dye, if macular edema is present.

3. HYPERTENSIVE RETINOPATHY

The general response of the arterial system of the body to hypertension is that of narrowing (autoregulation). The retinal arteriolar constriction in response to systemic hypertension is, however, modified by the degree and the extent of pre-existing involutional sclerosis in these vessels. Therefore, while a generalized narrowing of the retinal arterioles is seen in young hypertensives, the degree of narrowing seen in the older individuals is less marked and irregular on account of the rigidity of the vessels caused by the involutionary sclerosis.

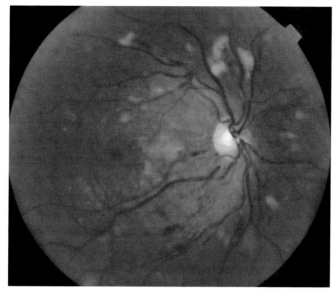

FIGURE 2.26: Hypertensive retinopathy
Generalized thickening (sclerosis) of retinal arteries, retinal hemorrhages, and several
cotton-wool spots resulting from the closure of precapillary arterioles

Vasoconstriction in the retina is seen in the form of generalized or focal narrowing of the arterioles. In severe hypertension, precapillary arterioles may show closure leading to the appearance of cotton-wool spots *(Figure 2.26)*.

Leakage from vessels, because of increased permeability, manifests in the form of flame-shaped retinal hemorrhages, hard exudates but, only a mild retinal edema. The hard exudates may collect around the macula in Henley's layer in a radiating, star-shaped fashion—*macular star.*

Arteriosclerosis causes thickening of the arterial wall on account of medial hyperplasia, and endothelial thickening. The effects of thickening are visible in the form of nipping of the veins at the arteriovenous (A-V) crossings.

Based on the fundus appearance, hypertensive retinopathy has been classified into four grades.

Grade 1. It shows in the form of mild, generalized narrowing, especially of the smaller branches. The arterial reflex is broadened along with concealment of the veins at the arteriovenous crossings.

Grade 2. It is characterized by a more severe, generalized and focal constriction of arterioles. There is deflection of the veins at the A-V crossings—*Salus' sign (Figure 2.27A).*

Grade 3. Further thickening of the vessel wall and narrowing cause the vessel to look like 'copper wire'. There is banking of veins distal to the A-V crossings (*Bonnet sign*). The arteries tend to cross the veins at right angles, and tapering of the veins is seen on either side of the A-V crossings—*Gunn sign (Figure 2.27B).* At this stage, flame-shaped hemorrhages, cotton-wool spots, and hard exudates are also seen.

Grade 4. In addition to the picture seen in grade 3 retinopathy, the arterioles look like thin white lines *(silver-wire' arteries)*, and swelling of the optic disk appears.

Fluorescein angiography (Figure 2.28) shows a generalized narrowing of the vessels, blocked fluorescence and capillary non-perfusion in areas corresponding to the retinal hemorrhages and cotton-wool spots, respectively. In the eyes with grade 4 retinopathy, edema of the optic disk causes dilated peripapillary capillaries and leakage of dye from the disk.

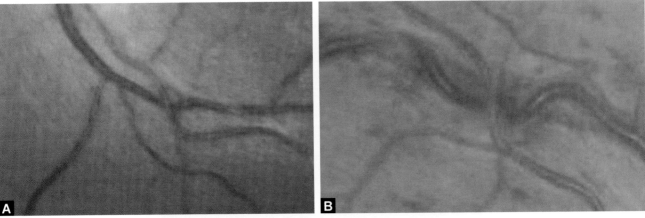

FIGURES 2.27A and B: Hypertensive retinopathy
A. Deflection of retinal vein at the arteriovenous crossing—Salus' sign
B. Banking of retinal vein distal to the arteriovenous crossing—Bonmet sign

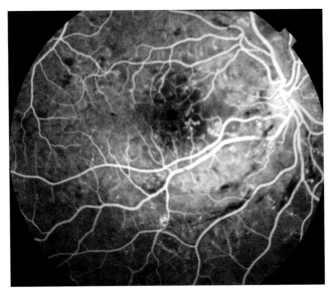

FIGURE 2.28: Hypertensive retinopathy
Angiogram shows blocked choroidal fluorescence due to retinal hemorrhages,
patches of NCP in the areas of cotton-wool spots

Treatment

It consists of the management of hypertension by the physician.

4. DIABETIC RETINOPATHY

Ophthalmic complications of diabetes include corneal abnormalities, glaucoma, iris neovascularization, cataracts and neuropathy. However, the most common, and potentially most blinding of these complications is diabetic retinopathy.

It is a microangiopathy involving the small vessels particularly in and around the macular area. The incidence of retinopathy is largely related to the duration of diabetes. About half the cases after 10 years of diabetes develop diabetic retinopathy. After 30 years of the disease, the incidence of diabetic retinopathy is nearly 90%.

It is rare to find diabetic retinopathy in cases with diabetes of less than 5 years' duration. The role of a good metabolic control of diabetes in the prevention of diabetic retinopathy is unequivocal. It may, perhaps, delay its development by a few years. Pregnancy, hypertension, and renal disease, and to some extent, smoking and obesity are the chief risk factors.

Growth hormone is believed to be the causative factor in the development and progression of diabetic retinopathy, being responsible for increased concentrations of high molecular weight proteins in the blood. It is supplemented by other hematological changes in the form of increased sedimentation rate, higher levels of hemoglobin A1c, rigidity (decreased deformability) of red blood cells, increased platelet aggregation and adhesion. Such changes predispose to sluggish circulation, endothelial damage, loss of pericytes, and focal capillary occlusions.

Another view suggests that the increased capillary permeability and macular edema is caused by shunting of excess glucose that increases the concentration of diacylglycerol (DAG). This, in turn, acts to activate protein kinase C (PKC) affecting the retinal blood dynamics, especially permeability and flow, responsible for fluid leakage and retinal thickening.

The basic factors in the development of diabetic retinopathy consist of (a) *increased capillary permeability* (causing *retinal edema and retinal hemorrhages*), and (b) *retinal hypoxia* (causing *neovascularization*).

The development of *macular edema* (diabetic maculopathy) is the most important factor responsible for visual loss in diabetic retinopathy. Visual loss due to macular edema is about 5 times the visual loss caused by the proliferative changes and its complications. Diabetic maculopathy is three times more common in non-insulin dependant diabetes (NIDDM) as compared with insulin dependent diabetes (IDDM). The maculopathy is best diagnosed by employing various binocular techniques of fundus examination (e.g. binocular indirect ophthalmoscopy with a 90 D lens and slit-lamp biomicroscopy with Goldmann's 3-mirror lens).

The state of *retinal hypoxia* results into *(i), arteriovenous shunts*, associated with a significant extent of capillary closure ('drop-out' or CNP). These vessels run from venules to arterioles *(Figures 2.29A and B)*, and are termed as 'intraretinal microvascular abnormalities' (IRMA); and *(ii), neovascularization* believed to be the result of certain growth factors (VEGF) liberated from the hypoxic retina, in an attempt to re-vascularize the hypoxic areas. The new vessels thus formed *(Figures 2.30A to I)* may be located in the retinal zone-NVE, or on the optic disk-NVD and later on, in the iris (NVI).

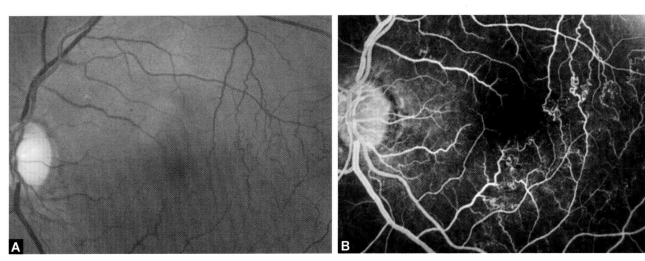

FIGURES 2.29A and B: Diabetic retinopathy
Shunt vessels (IRMA) in diabetic retinopathy

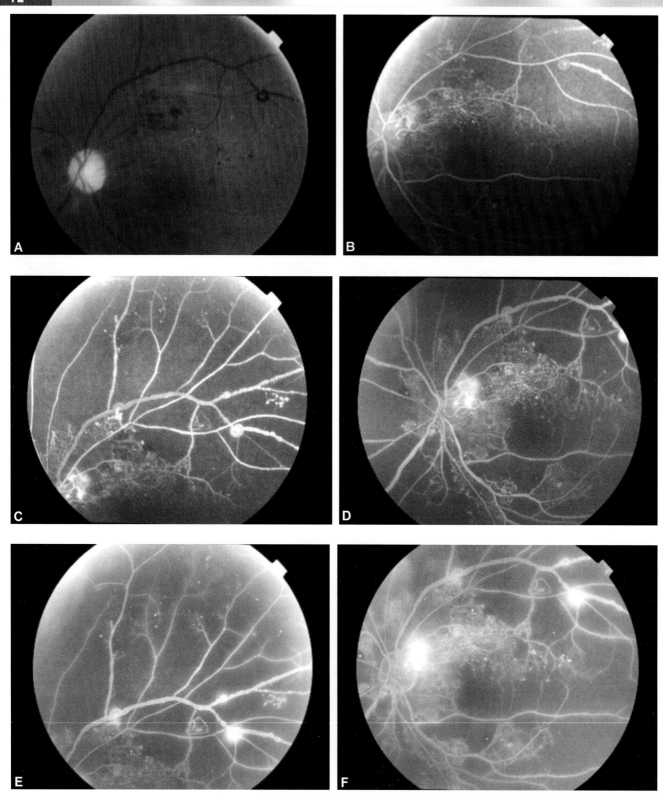

FIGURES 2.30A to F: Diabetic retinopathy
PDR, the serial angiogram shows wide spread areas of NCP, and hyperfluorescence on the disk
and elsewhere on the retina caused by NVD and NVE respectively

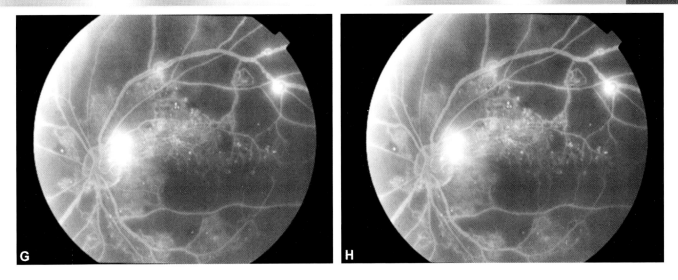

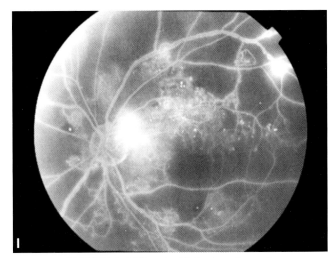

FIGURES 2.30G to I: Diabetic retinopathy
PDR, the serial angiogram shows wide spread areas of NCP, and hyperfluorescence on the disk
and elsewhere on the retina caused by NVD and NVE respectively

Classification

Clinically, diabetic retinopathy is classified as:
  A. Non-proliferative diabetic retinopathy, and
  B. Proliferative diabetic retinopathy.

Non-proliferative Diabetic Retinopathy

Non-proliferative diabetic retinopathy is characterized by the presence of microaneurysms; retinal hemorrhages, hard exudates, and retinal edema *(Figure 2.31).*

Microaneurysms are amongst the first clinically detectable signs of diabetic retinopathy. They appear as small round dots, usually located temporal to the macula. Because of the increased permeability and the weakened wall as a result of the loss of pericytes, they contribute to cause retinal edema and retinal hemorrhages.

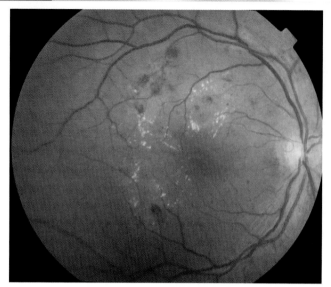

FIGURE 2.31: Diabetic retinopathy
NPDR with microaneurysms, retinal hemorrhages, hard
exudates and retinal edema

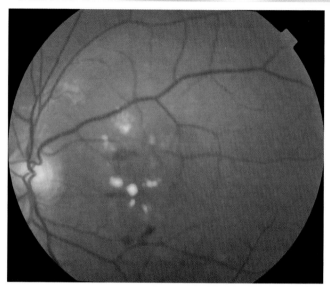

FIGURE 2.32: Diabetic retinopathy
Clinically significant macular edema

Retinal hemorrhages may be superficial ('flame shaped') or deep ('dot-blot)' hemorrhages. The flame-shaped hemorrhages originate from the superficial precapillary arterioles and spread along the fibers of the nerve-fiber layer. The dot-blot hemorrhages originate from the venous end of the capillaries and lie within the compact deeper layers of the retina.

Hard exudates are small yellow and waxy looking spots with relatively diskrete margins, arranged in clumps and/or rings (around a central microaneurysm), and located mostly at the posterior pole. They tend to increase in size and number, with time.

Retinal edema at the macula starts between the outer plexiform and the inner nuclear layer of the retina, followed by the collection of fluid in the inner nuclear layer and nerve-fiber layer, ultimately involving the full retinal thickness. Further increase in edema may lead to the formation of cystoid spaces—*cystoid macular edema.*

Edema at the macula is termed *clinically significant macular edema (CSME) (Figure 2.32)* in the presence of one or more of the following features:
- Retinal edema within 500 micron of the fovea.
- Hard exudates within 500 micron of the fovea with adjacent retinal thickening.
- Retinal edema that is one disk area or larger, any part of which is within 1 disk diameter of the center of fovea.

CSME is called *focal macular edema* that is associated with hard exudate rings resulting from leakage from microaneurysms *(Figures 2.33A and B). Diffuse macular edema,* on the other hand, results from breakdown of blood-retinal barrier with leakage from microaneurysms, retinal capillaries, and arterioles *(Figures 2.34A and B).*

Based on the severity of various features, non-proliferative diabetic retinopathy (NPDR) is graded as *mild, moderate, severe* and *very severe type.*

Mild NPDR
- Presence of at least one microaneurysm.
- Fifteen percent of such eyes are likely to develop high risk PDR in 5 years.

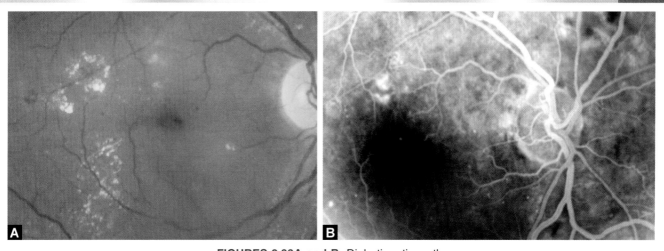

FIGURES 2.33A and B: Diabetic retinopathy
A. Focal macular edema
B. Angiogram of focal macular edema shows focal area of leakage from the upper part of macula

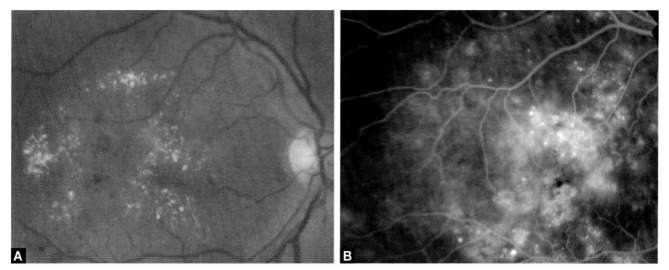

FIGURES 2.34A and B: Diabetic retinopathy
A. Diffuse macular edema
B. Angiogram showing diffuse leakage of dye at the macula

Moderate NPDR
- Presence of microaneurysms, hemorrhages, and hard exudates or,
- Presence of few soft exudates, mild venous beading and IRMA.
- Likelihood of developing features of high risk PDR are 3% in one year and 27% in 5 years.

Severe NPDR (4-2-1)
- Hemorrhages and exudates in all the four quadrants or,
- Venous beading in at least 2 quadrants or,
- IRMA in at least one quadrant.
- Risk of developing severe PDR in 15% eyes after 1 year; 27% after 5 years.

Very severe NPDR. Any of the two or more features of severe NPDR. Nearly half the eyes are likely to develop high risk PDR in one year and nearly three quarters in 5 years.

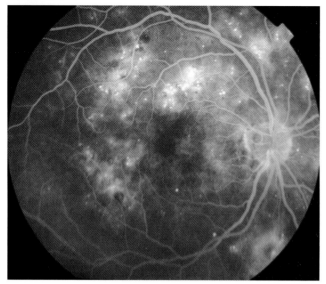

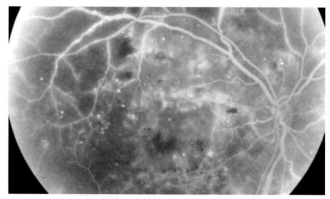

FIGURE 2.36: Diabetic retinopathy
NPDR with areas of NCP

FIGURE 2.35: Diabetic retinopathy
Angiogram of NPDR shows patches of hypofluorescence due
to retinal hemorrhage; hyperfluorescent areas are due to
leakage of dye from microaneurysms

Fundus fluorescein angiography (Figure 2.35) shows
microaneurysms as fluorescent dots. Patchy areas of
blocked fluorescence are caused by the superficial and deep
hemorrhages. Leakage of dye from the microaneurysms
appears as areas of hyperfluorescence. Capillary closure is
seen as areas of hypofluorescence that are usually bordered
by dilated capillaries and microaneurysms *(Figure 2.36)*.
IRMA are seen as vessels crossing the horizontal raphe,
originating from venules. These vessels do not leak
fluorescein *(Figures 2.29A and B)*.

Treatment is indicated if CSME is present. Based on the
fluorescein angiographic picture, it consists of a focal laser
coagulation of isolated points of leakage
(Figures 2.33A and B), or grid-pattern coagulation in eyes
with a diffuse leakage *(Figures 2.34A and B)*. No
coagulation is considered in eyes with an ischemic

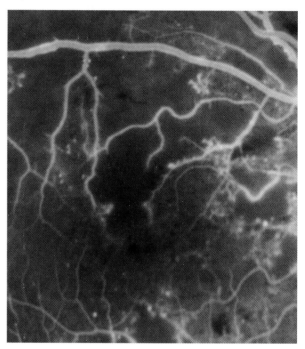

FIGURE 2.37: Diabetic retinopathy
Ischemic maculopathy in a case of PDR

maculopathy *(Figure 2.37)* that have a poor prognosis. Intravitreal injection of steroids and anti-VEGF drugs
(as described in the treatment of wet ARMD) have shown encouraging results in the treatment of diabetic
macular edema, as well as that of new vessel formation.

Periodic assessment of the retinal condition is necessary. In cases with mild NPDR without retinal edema,
recheck is advised yearly, but more frequently (every 3 to 6 months) in cases with more severe forms of
retinopathy. Similarly, in cases with macular edema (CSME or Non-CSME) fundus examination is carried out
more frequently (every 2-4 months).

Proliferative Diabetic Retinopathy (PDR)

Proliferative diabetic retinopathy (PDR) is seen in 5-10% cases of the diabetic population. Patients with IDDM
are at a greater risk than those with NIDDM.

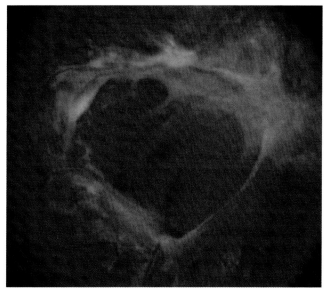

FIGURE 2.43: Diabetic retinopathy
TRD in PDR

The new vessels are initially associated with a small amount of fibroglial tissue that increases with the increase in the size of neovascular frond. In the late stages the blood vessels may regress leaving behind a network of fibroglial tissue. This exerts traction and may lead to retinal detachment *(Figure 2.43)* with or without a retinal tear.

The following features of the disease are considered as *high-risk characteristics*:
1. NVD of more than 1/4 disk area in size.
2. NVD with pre-retinal or vitreous hemorrhage.
3. NVE of at least 1/2 disk area in extent with pre-retinal or vitreous hemorrhage.

Fundus fluorescein angiography (Figure 2.44) reveals, in addition to the changes visible in non-proliferative diabetic retinopathy, large areas of NCP and new vessel formation (NVE, NVD, or both). Leakage of dye from the new vessels manifests as hyperfluorescence.

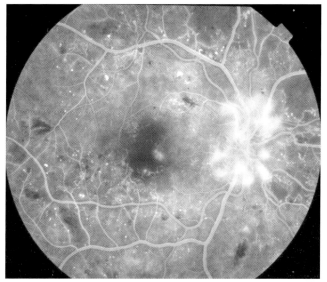

FIGURE 2.44: Diabetic retinopathy
Angiogram of PDR showing NCP, NVD, and ischemic maculopathy

Treatment. The aim of all forms of therapy proposed to treat proliferative diabetic retinopathy is primarily to arrest the progress of the disease and to maintain and improve the visual acuity to the maximum possible extent.

Medical, intensive glucose control, according to the perspective clinical trial (DCCT), in patients with insulin-dependent diabetes mellitus (IDDM) decreased the incidence as well as the progression of diabetic retinopathy. Although no similar trials have been made in the case of non-insulin dependent diabetes mellitus, it may be logically assumed that the principles apply.

In a recent phase III trial, intravitreal injections of bovine hyaluronidase have been shown to be safe and materially effective in clearing of dense vitreous hemorrhage.

More recently, Avastin has been used to treat vitreous hemorrhage. In addition, this medicine has been used to treat optic nerve or retinal neovascularization as well as rubeosis.

Laser treatment is one of the mainstays for the treatment of diabetic retinopathy. This form of treatment has a relatively low complication rate and a significant degree of success.

While a focal or sectorial coagulation is required in most eyes of NPDR, pan-retinal photocoagulation (PRP) is the preferred form of treatment for PDR. Delivery systems for the treatment include slit-lamp microscope, indirect ophthalmoscope, and the EndoProbe. General guidelines for the indication of laser coagulation treatment are as follows:
1. Clinically significant macular edema (CSME), irrespective of the grade of retinopathy.
2. Severe/very severe NPDR (treatment with full scatter-PRP along with appropriate management of CSME).
3. Evidence of high-risk characters (PRP).

The treatment may be undertaken in earlier stages in certain situations such as:
*   Monocular patients
*   Non-compliant patients
*   Pregnancy
*   Inadequate eye care facility
*   Hypertension/subnormal renal function.

The following protocol is recommended for treating diabetic retinopathy with laser photocoagulation:
*   Total number of 1,200-1,600 applications of 200-500 micron size (gray-white burns) is made, one burn spot size apart in two or three sessions. The areas of new vessels are spared.
*   Presence of high-risk PDR is an indication for immediate treatment.
*   In cases where macular edema and PDR co-exist, laser treatments are performed, first for the macular edema, and the PRP is spread over 3-4 sessions. If it is necessary to treat them together, the PRP is affected initially on the nasal third of the retina.
*   The strategy of treating macular edema depends on the type and extent of vessel leakage. If the edema is due to focal leakage, microaneurysms are treated directly. In cases where the foci of leakage are non-specific, a grid pattern of laser is applied. Burns of 100-200 micron size are placed, one burn apart, covering the affected area.

The exact mechanism by which PRP works is not entirely understood. According to one theory, destroying the hypoxic retina presumably reduces the liberation of vasoproliferative factors such as VEGF that in turn reduces the rate of neovascularization. Another theory is that PRP allows increased diffusion of oxygen from the choroid, supplementing retinal circulation. The enhanced oxygenation also reduces the liberation of vaso-proliferative factors and subsequent vasoproliferation.

Vitrectomy may be necessary mainly in cases of longstanding vitreous hemorrhage (with or without rubeosis), tractional retinal detachment, and combined tractional and rhegmatogenous retinal detachment. The Diabetic Retinopathy Vitrectomy Study (DRVS) has recommended that vitrectomy be advised for eyes with vitreous hemorrhage that fails to resolve spontaneously within 6 months. Monitoring of cases with ultrasonography is necessary for all cases of delayed vitrectomy. However, an early vitrectomy may be indicated in the following situations:

- IDDM patients with severe vitreous hemorrhage of one-month duration.
- Patients with vitreous hemorrhage having poor vision in the other eye.
- Patients with active and advanced PDR (even with an adequate visual acuity) where an adequate laser treatment has failed to affect any significant regression of the new vessels.
- Patients with active and advanced PDR, where the presence of vitreous hemorrhage prevents laser treatment.
- Patients with neovascularization of the iris (NVI) of more than 2 clock hours in extent
- Patients with a tractional retinal detachment (TRD) involving the macula.

The purpose of surgery is to remove the blood for visualization of the posterior segment to plan the subsequent treatment; to release tractional forces pulling on the retina; to repair retinal detachment, and to remove the scaffolding into which the fibrovascular tissue may grow. In addition, vitrectomy provides the opportunity for the initiation of PRP through EndoProbe or indirect ophthalmoscope.

Cryopexy. Laser photocoagulation of retina may not be possible in eyes with opaque media such as cataract or vitreous hemorrhage. In these circumstances cryotherapy may be used for retinal coagulation.

5. COATS' DISEASE

Coats' Disease. (Syn. Exudative Retinitis; Retinal Telangiectasis). Coats' disease is a condition (or perhaps, a group of conditions) with the common characteristics of massive retinal and subretinal exudation along with vascular malformations of various kinds. Two clinical forms have been described—*juvenile* and *adult* form. The juvenile form is much more common, and is seen in young individuals (8-16 years, sometimes younger), predominantly males. The disease is unilateral in over 80% of cases, affecting healthy individuals with no evidence of any hereditary background. The pathogenesis is not clearly understood. It may be caused by a functional or structural breakdown of the blood-retinal barrier of obscure origin. Due to capillary closure at the telengiectasia, retinal neovascularization with subsequent vitreous hemorrhage and tractional retinal detachment can occur. Current research suggests a genetic component contributing to the disease by locating the disease gene on the short arm (p) of the X-chromosome (Xp 11.4). Accordingly, the patient is born with the disease, without being hereditary in nature. The symptoms and the progress of the disease depend on the number and the size of the blood vessels involved.

In children the disease is recognized because of the complaint of poor vision, strabismus, or appearance of leukokoria. Fundus examination reveals characteristic large areas of raised dirty-yellow looking exudates over and under the retina in the central retina, which mask the visualization of the retinal vessels *(Figures 2.45 and 2.46A)*. Glistening spots or areas, suggestive of cholesterol deposits are usually present. Retinal detachment is of common occurrence and the retina may be pushed far forwards behind the lens causing the appearance of leukokoria. The exudative process is progressive (with periods of remissions) and leads to iridocyclitis, complicated cataract, secondary glaucoma and eventually phthisis bulbi. Young children do not appreciate the symptoms and thus, may be unaware of the disease. One early sign of Coats' disease is 'yellow eye' in flash photography.

The retinal vascular anomalies which are responsible for the exudation, occur in small clusters localized to a few vessels, or grouped over all sectors of the retina. The vascular anomalies consist of tortuous, looped or kinked vessels with perivascular sheathing. Some vessels may show aneurysmal dilatations with saccular and sausage-shaped swellings. The vascular abnormalities and exudation show a predilection for the temporal retina. Exudation in the macular area is seen even when the vascular abnormalities are located remotely in the more peripheral zone.

The adult form of Coats' disease runs relatively a milder course as compared to the juvenile form. The adult patients may show high levels of serum cholesterol, which is not the case in the juvenile variety.

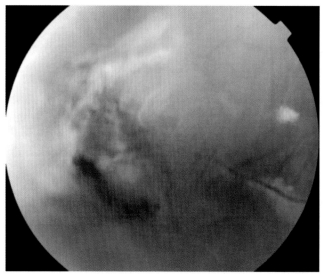

FIGURE 2.45: Coats' disease
Massive exudation and hemorrhage in an advanced case of Coats' disease

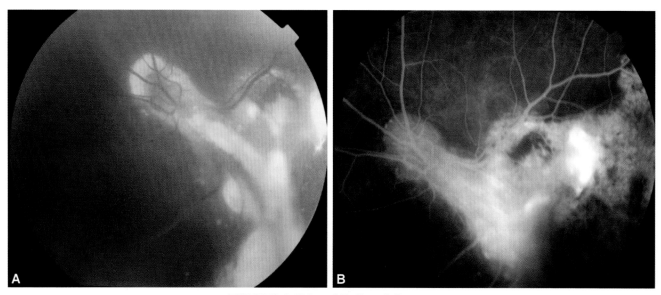

FIGURES 2.46A and B: Coats' disease
A. Massive exudation with abnormal vessel
B. Angiogram shows leakage of dye and staining of the scar tissue

Fundus fluorescein angiography. Fluorescein angiogram shows localized vascular anomalies. Late films show leakage of dye *(Figure 2.46B).*

Treatment

Treatment in children is usually extremely difficult, and mostly, unrewarding. It consists of coagulation of the abnormal vessels with cryotherapy, laser or xenon photocoagulation that may be effective only in early cases having localized vascular anomalies with mild-to-moderate exudation.

Surgery to repair retinal detachment may be required in some cases. Vitrectomy is often necessary during the procedure.

Chapter

(3)

Inflammations

1. ACUTE MULTIFOCAL POSTERIOR PIGMENT EPITHELIOPATHY (AMPPE)

AMPPE is an acquired inflammatory disorder affecting the retina, retinal pigment epithelium and the choroid. Its pathogenesis is speculative, but the basic underlying mechanism is believed to be an obstructive vasculitis causing non-perfusion of the terminal globules at the posterior pole of choroid, inducing secondary ischemic injury to the retinal pigment epithelium and the photoreceptors. It is further believed that the ocular manifestation is a part of diffuse multisystem vasculitis. Systemic involvement though uncommon, may include erythema nodosum, thyroiditis, microvascular nephropathy, and neurological manifestations like cerebral vasculitis, transient ischemic attacks, vertigo, etc. Higher frequency of human leukocyte antigens B7 (HLA-B7) and HLA-DR2 have been reported, suggesting an inherited tendency for the disorder.

In the acute phase, the disease is characterized by appearance of multiple, subretinal, placoid, yellow-white lesions in both eyes *(Figure 3.1)*. If unilateral, the other eye may be involved within a short period. The onset of the disease is preceded by flu-like ailment in about a third of case. New lesions may appear in the affected eye as the older lesions begin resolution. Rarely, a well-demarcated serous detachment of retina may be present *(Figure 3.2)*. Hyperemia of optic disk and blurring of disk margins along with engorgement of retinal veins may be present. Occurrence of papillitis and optic neuritis is rare. Mild vitritis is present in about half the cases. The patient complains of acute or subacute decrease in vision that is generally mild in nature. Photopsia, metmorphopsia or micropsia may also be present.

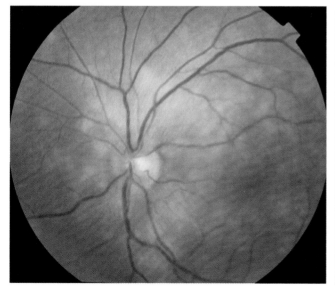

FIGURE 3.1: AMPPE
Multiple, subretinal, placoid, yellow-white lesions

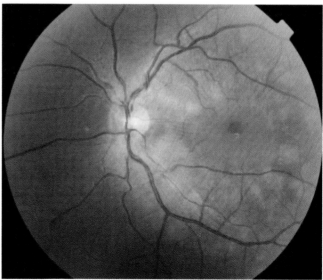

FIGURE 3.2: AMPPE
Lesions of AMPPE with detachment of sensory retina
at the macula

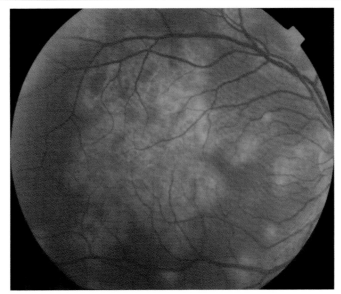

FIGURE 3.3: AMPPE
Recurrent AMPPE; fresh lesions along with the healed lesions

In late stages of the disease, mild visual impairment may remain. Significant visual loss is rare. Resolution of the lesion takes the form of well-demarcatd areas of RPE loss with fine foci of hyperplasia. Long-term follow-up suggests that recurrence may develop in 50% cases *(Figure 3.3)*.

AMPPE may be complicated, though rarely, by choroidal neovascularization and retinal vein thrombosis. Death has been reported in case of severe cerebral vasculitis.

AMPPE is diagnosed by its typical clinical appearance and disease course. No test is diagnostic or pathognomonic of the disease. On *fundus fluorescein angiography,* early lesions exhibit hypofluorescence, followed by hyperfluorescence with or without staining *(Figures 3.4A and B).* Older lesions show window

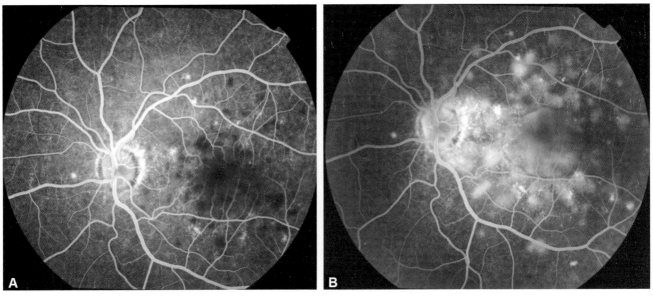

FIGURES 3.4A and B: AMPPE
Angiogram shows spot of hypofluorescence in early phase A, and hyperfluorescence in the later phases B

defects in RPE. CT/MRI is indicated rarely in case with severe headache or CNS symptoms. Cerebral angiogram may be required in cases of suspected cerebral vasculitis.

Treatment

AMPPE is a self-limiting disease requiring no treatment. A short course of systemic steroids has been suggested in cases with macular involvement.

2. ACUTE MULTIFOCAL CHOROIDITIS

Acute multifocal choroiditis (AMC) affects young, healthy individuals (women more than men), commonly in the third decade of life, and is mostly bilateral.

The usual presenting symptoms are blurring of vision, floaters, metamorphopsia, and photopsia. Visual loss may vary from mild to severe, with an average visual acuity of 6/36. Nearly half of the cases show anterior chamber reaction in the form of mild-to-moderate degree of flare and cells. Small and intermediate-sized keratic precipitates may be present. Vitreous cellular infiltrates are present in 90% cases.

Fundus examination reveals multiple, small to medium sized, discrete, pale-yellow spots that are mostly round in shape *(Figure 3.5)*. The lesions tend to be present in the mid-periphery, sparing the macula. Some patients may have optic disk edema. During the late stage of the disease, the spots become atrophic with a variable degree of hyperpigmentation at the borders. Recurrences are common.

Complications of cystoid macular edema (CME) has been reported in 10-20% cases, and appearance of choroidal neovascularization (CNV) in nearly one-third of cases.

The etiology of AMC remains, largely unknown. Extensive systemic evaluation and laboratory investigations have failed to determine the cause of the disease. However, tubercular infection has been suspected to be associated, in 20% cases because of radiological evidence of hilar lymphadenitis and positive skin reaction to tuberculin, and therapeutic response to anti-tubercular therapy. Sarcoidosis has also been implied in several cases. Other infections that have been associated with AMC are herpes simplex, herpes zoster, Epstein-Barr virus, and toxocara canis. Despite these reports, many investigators believe that AMC results from an underlying autoimmune mechanism, possibly triggered by an infective agent.

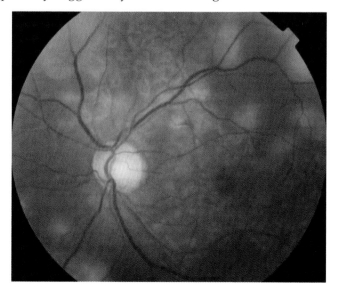

FIGURE 3.5: Acute multifocal choroiditis
Medium sized, round, yellow spots in the mid-periphery;
healed, pigmented lesions are visible centrally

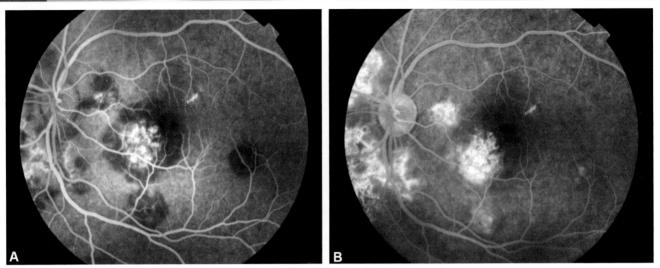

FIGURES 3.6A and B: Acute multifocal choroiditis
Angiogram shows hypofluorescence in the early phase A, and hyperfluorescence in the later phases B

Visual prognosis is variable, being usually poor in recurrent cases. The major cause or the severe visual loss is the development of CNV, and to a lesser extent due to CME. Approximately one-third cases maintain the visual acuity at onset, while another one-third lose two or more Snellen lines.

Fundus fluorescein angiography. Early pictures show hypofluorescence corresponding to the lesion followed by hyperfluorescence *(Figures 3.6A and B)*.

Treatment

In the acute phase of the disease, several cases show a prompt response to high doses of systemic corticosteroids, with subsequent improvement of vision. However, with each recurrence, the affectivity of steroids is reduced.

Immunomodulatory therapy with azathiopurine, cyclosporine, and methotrexate, often show good control of the disease, and in the subsequent preservation of vision.

CNV is managed with conventional lasers, photodynamic therapy (PDT), or with the help of emerging treatment with VEGF-inhibitors such as mucogen, lucentis, and avastin.

3. GEOGRAPHIC HELICOID PERIPAPILLARY CHOROIDOPATHY (GHPC)

Also called *serpiginous choroidopathy*, it is an uncommon bilateral, chronic and progressive inflammation of the retinal pigment epithelium and the inner choroid, typically seen between the forth and sixth decade of life, in both sexes. It usually starts with a reduction in visual acuity in one eye, the other being involved after a variable period. The visual prognosis is generally bad.

The lesion typically arises from the peripapillary region and spreads centrifugally in pseudopod or geographic fashion. Unfortunately, the condition has a predilection for the temporal rather than the nasal retina. Choroidal vascularization develops in 25% cases. Occasionally, it is associated with retinal periphlebitis, branch retinal vein occlusion, and detachment of retinal pigment epithelium.

Retinal examination reveals the presence of cream-colored patches with hazy borders located near the disk *(Figure 3.7)*. They spread in all directions involving also, the macular area resulting in a profound and permanent visual loss. Mild anterior uveitis and vitritis may be present. Spontaneous healing takes place in the form of pale white punched out scars with densely pigmented margins. Fresh crops of lesions appear leading to widespread scarring that has irregular snake-like borders.

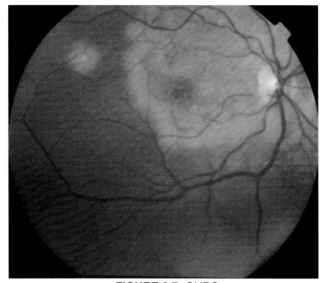

FIGURE 3.7: GHPC
Cream-colored patch with hazy borders adjoining the optic disk, an isolated lesion is also seen

Etiology of GHPC remains elusive. Histological studies reveal that it is a non-granulomatous choroiditis. Immunologic mechanism is suspected by its association with human leukocyte antigens A2 (HLA-A2) and B7 (HLA-B7) histocompatibility.

On *FFA*, active lesions show hypofluorescence in the early phases, and staining in the late films *(Figure 3.8)*.

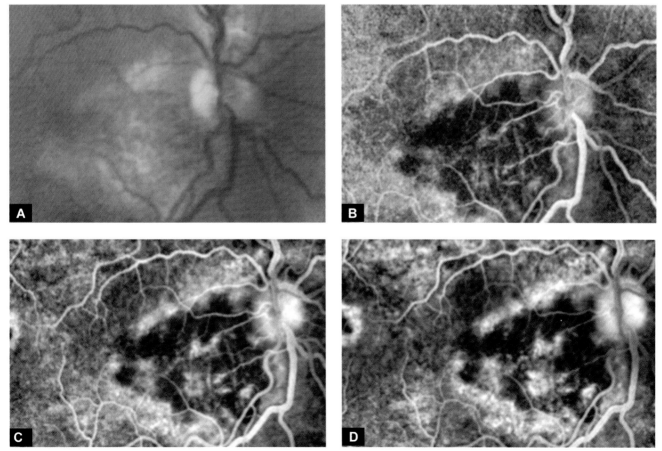

FIGURES 3.8A to D

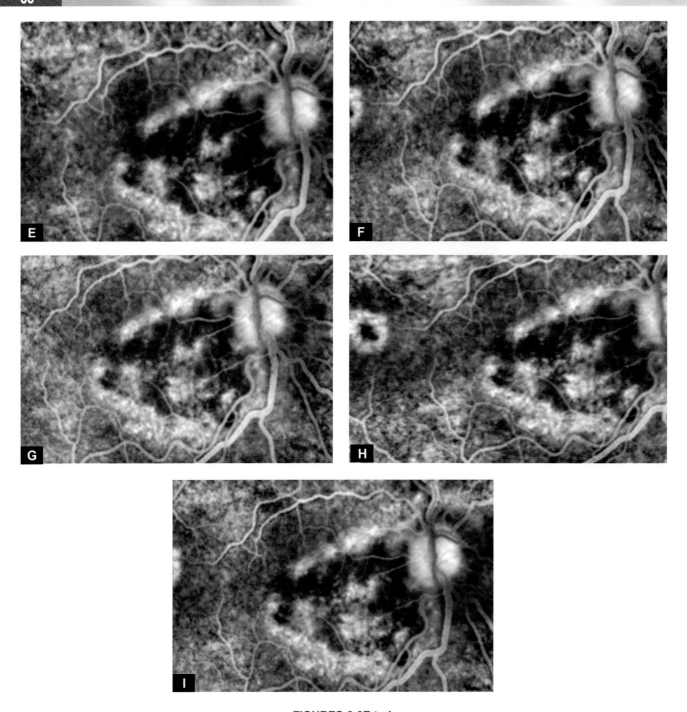

FIGURES 3.8E to I
FIGURES A to I: GHPC
Serial angiogram shows hypofluorescence in the early phase and staining in the late phase

Treatment

Systemic steroids and cytotoxic drugs (cyclosporine, azathiopurine) are used with uncertain results. CNVM, if present, is treated with the recommended procedures.

4. TOXOPLASMIC RETINOCHOROIDITIS

A toxoplasmic lesion in the retina, generally seen between the ages of 10 to 30 years, is believed to be nearly always the result of recurrence of a healed congenital lesion. In congenital toxoplasmosis, the disease is passed on to the fetus through the placenta, if the mother happens to receive infection during pregnancy. A pre-natal infection does not affect the child. Likewise, a woman with a child having evidence of congenital toxoplasmosis, will not have the subsequent children born with the disease.

Toxoplasma infection during early pregnancy causes stillbirth, or the child is born with widespread involvement, especially that of the central nervous system. In the case of a milder infection during the third trimester in a woman with normal immune system, the born child may be normal and asymptomatic. The retinal lesion, if present, may be discovered incidentally on fundus examination. It appears a punched out white scar with hyperpigmented margins. If located at the macula, it resembles a macular coloboma *(Figure 3.9)*.

The retinal involvement is seen in the form of usually a single, or occasionally, multiple necrotizing white lesions with surrounding retinal edema and vitreous haze. The lesions are located commonly in the post-equatorial retina, adjacent to the scar of a congenital lesion *(Figures 3.10A and B)*. These lesions are caused by the liberation of bacteria from the cysts persisting in the healed lesion. Nearly half of the eyes show recurrences at the average rate of 3 recurrences per eye.

The patient may complain of visual haze if the lesion is placed peripherally and is accompanied by only a mild vitritis. More commonly, vitreous haze is dense causing a significant fogginess of vision. Lesions located at or around the macula, papillomacular bundle, or the optic nerve head cause a profound visual loss. A mild to moderate iridocyclitis is usually present. These lesions gradually heal in 2-3 month's time giving rise to scar formation.

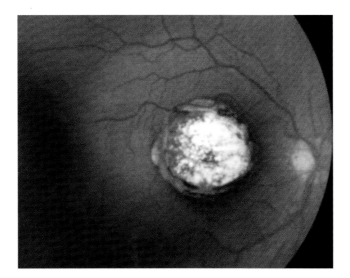

FIGURE 3.9: Toxoplasmosis
Healed lesion of congenital toxoplasmosis, simulating congenital coloboma of macula

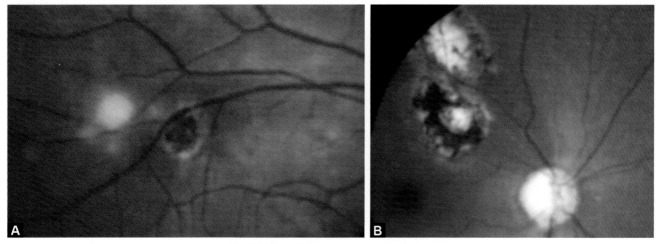

FIGURES 3.10A and B: Toxoplasmosis
A. Lesion of acute toxoplasmosis adjoining the healed lesion, B. Healed lesions of toxoplasmosis

Treatment

Treatment is indicated if the lesion is threatening or involving the macula, papillomacular bundle, optic nerve or a major blood vessel; or in cases with a severe vitritis causing a considerable loss of vision. However, all types of lesions in an immunodeficient person need treatment.

Administration of systemic steroids is a constant part of treatment. No definite advantage has been seen when additional drugs (pyrimethamine, co-trimexazole, clindamycin and other antibiotics) are added to steroids, though the recurrence rate may perhaps, be reduced.

5. EALES' DISEASE (PERIPHLEBITIS RETINAE)

Eales' Disease (Periphlebitis Retinae). Primary retinal periphlebitis is the most common form of retinal vasculitis, frequently seen in the subcontinent. The disease is of unknown etiology although several factors such as tuberculosis, sarcoidosis, syphilis, immune reactions, etc. have been suggested from time to time as the underlying factors.

The disease, most commonly, affects young adults, predominantly males. In the initial stage of the disease the patient may be asymptomatic, or the patient may complain of floaters and visual haze. Later on, these symptoms may be exaggerated and in addition, marked loss of vision of sudden occurrence, may take place indicating a vitreous hemorrhage. Such episodes of vitreous hemorrhage causing sudden loss of vision may recur. In uncontrolled cases, permanent loss of vision may result, accompanied by a painful eye.

Basically, it is a vasoproliferative disease starting as an inflammation of the small peripheral vessels, predominantly the venules. Clinically, it manifests in the form of retinal edema and small retinal hemorrhages around the inflamed vessels, which may show cuffing at places *(Figures 3.11A and B)*. Healing takes place in the form of disappearance of retinal edema and hemorrhages. The affected veins, however, become narrower and appear strangulated by the perivascular sheathing *(Figure 3.12)*. The disease may start afresh in the same or some other sector. Gradually, the larger, posteriorly placed veins may get involved, which may on rare occasions, cause occlusion of these vessels *(Figure 3.13)*. The incompetence of the inflamed venules causes retinal hemorrhages, which may break through into the vitreous leading to a gross reduction in the visual acuity.

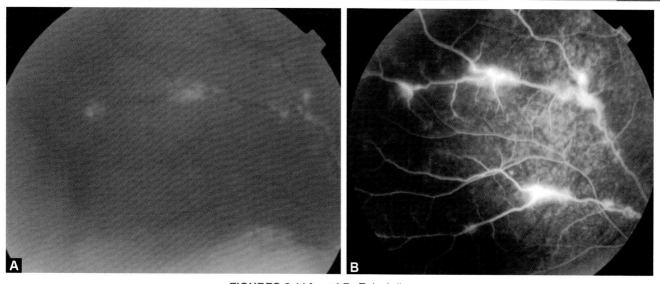

FIGURES 3.11A and B: Eales' disease

A. Acute stage of Eales' disease with exudation and small hemorrhages around the affected venules; B. Angiogram shows leakage of dye from the venules; staining of the affected venules; small patches of hypofluorescence around the vessels caused by small hemorrhages

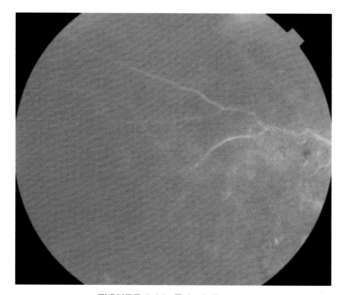

FIGURE 3.12: Eales' disease
Healed periphlebitis with perivascular sheathing
of the narrowed veins

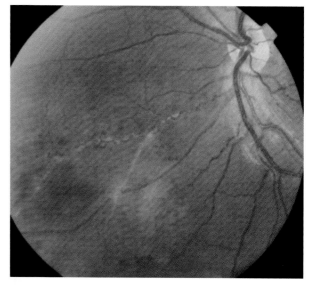

FIGURE 3.13: Eales' disease
Occlusive involvement of a large vein extending
posteriorly up to the optic disk

The vascular inflammation along with the endothelial proliferation and reduction in the caliber of these venules on account of the perivascular fibrous tissue, cause closure of the vessels leading to ischemia, manifesting as non-perfusion of retinal capillaries *(Figure 3.14)*. The state of hypoxia so produced, stimulates the release of vasoproliferative factor resulting in the proliferation of new blood vessels in the form of NVE *(Figure 3.15)*, NVD, or both *(Figures 3.16A and B)*.

Persistence of neovascularization is also responsible for repeated episodes of retinal and vitreous hemorrhages, which may cause formation of fibrous tissue on the retina that grows into the vitreous

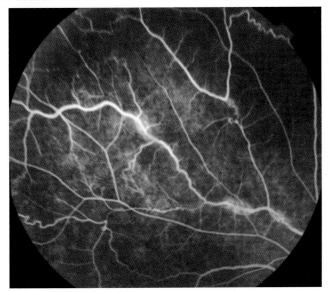

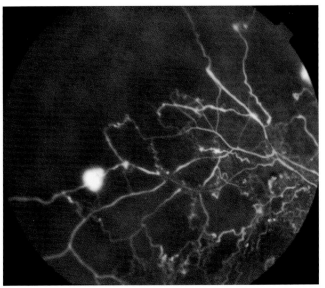

FIGURE 3.14: Eales' disease
Angiogram of healed disease shows narrowed veins,
staining of veins, IRMA, and NCP

FIGURE 3.15: Eales' disease
Angiogram of healed disease with large areas
of NCP leading to NVE

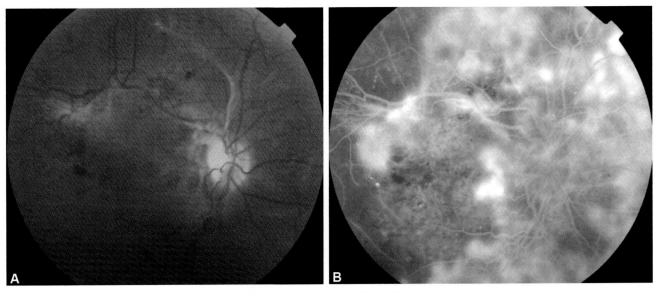

FIGURES 3.16A and B: Eales disease
A. Development of NVE and NVD following retinal ischemia in healed periphlebitis B. Angiogram shows extensive areas of hyperfluorescence caused by the leakage of fluorescein from the new vessel formations on the optic disk and elsewhere on the retina

(Figures 3.17 and 3.18). Traction on the retina as the result of fibrous tissue growth in the vitreous may lead to tractional retinal detachment (TRD) *(Figure 3.19).* In the advanced stage of ischemia, new vessel growth may invade the iris (NVI) causing intractable secondary rise in intraocular pressure [Neovascular glaucoma (NVG)]. The lens gets opaque (complicated cataract). The eye becomes painful due to NVG.

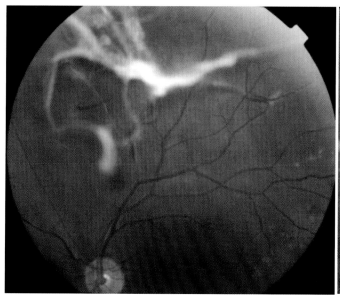

FIGURE 3.17: Eales' disease
Glial tissue proliferation in the retinal periphery

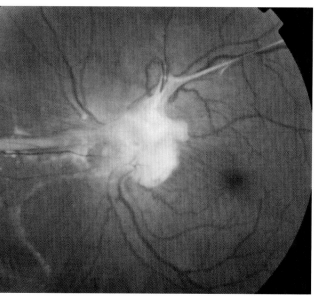

FIGURE 3.18: Eales' disease
Glial tissue proliferation over the optic disk, extending
peripherally over the retina

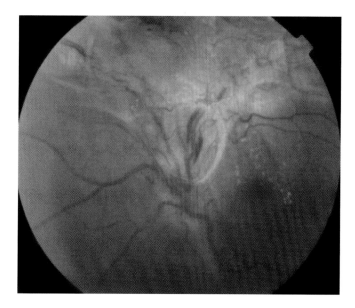

FIGURE 3.19: Eales' disease: Massive fibrovascular
proliferation causing tractional retinal detachment

Treatment

No specific treatment is available, though the administration of anti-tubercular drugs has been suggested. Anti-inflamatory drugs in the form of systemic corticosteroids have been recommended in the active phases. Administration of anti-oxidant vitamins A, C and E has been suggested on the basis of laboratory finding of deficient levels of these agents in the vitreous samples of patients with Eales' disease. An increased level of oxydation and peroxydation products was also observed in these samples. In the cases complicated with cystoid macular edema, intravitreal triamcinolone (2-4 mg) has been effective in reducing the edema and improving visual acuity. The use of certain *anti-VEGF agents* has been suggested that provides an exciting prospect meriting further investigation.

Laser coagulation is the chief form of treatment to prevent the complications caused by the vaso-proliferative component of the disease. In the case of localized areas of capillary non-perfusion with NVE, coagulation localized to these areas is effective in the obliteration of new vessels. Panretinal coagulation (PRP) is indicated in eyes with NVD, multiple areas of NVE, or in the eyes with extensive areas of NCP. The cases need to be followed up as new areas of neovascularization may develop.

Vitreoretinal surgery is required for cases with non-absorbing vitreous hemorrhage, or when a tractional retinal detachment is present. It may also be considered in eyes with recurrent vitreous hemorrhages where the vitreous cavity does not sufficiently clear up for a proper evaluation of the disease, in between the recurrences. After clearing of the vitreous cavity, laser coagulation has to follow in the manner as may be decided on the basis of fluorescein angiographic patterns.

Non-invasive procedures like laser/cryocoagulation of the ciliary body are employed for the control of neo-vascular glaucoma and pain.

6. SARCOIDOSIS

Sarcoidosis is a systemic, granulomatous disease of unknown etiology affecting several body organs singly, or in combination. The commonly affected organs include the lungs, skin, central nervous system and eyes. Racial predilection of the disease is well documented, affecting the American Black population much more frequently than the Whites. The acute form of the disease usually occurs in the third decade.

Ocular involvement is seen in nearly one-third cases of systemic sarcoidosis. The ocular surface lesions may involve the conjunctiva, episclera and, rarely, the sclera. Keratoconjunctivitis sicca may be seen in cases with involvement of lacrimal gland. The corneal stroma may be involved with a focal, avascular keratits (nummular keratitis).

Chronic granulomatous iridocyclitis is seen in older patients during the period when the systemic disease is inactive. It is characterized by the presence of minimal ciliary congestion, large mutton-fat keratic precipitates and nodules on the iris (Busacca nodules). The inflammation is often, difficult to control leading to complications such as cataract formation, secondary glaucoma and band keratopathy.

The posterior segment involvement is in the form of vitritis with cells and 'cotton ball' opacities located in the pre-retinal area, usually in the lower periphery. Periphlebitis is the most common form of retinal involvement

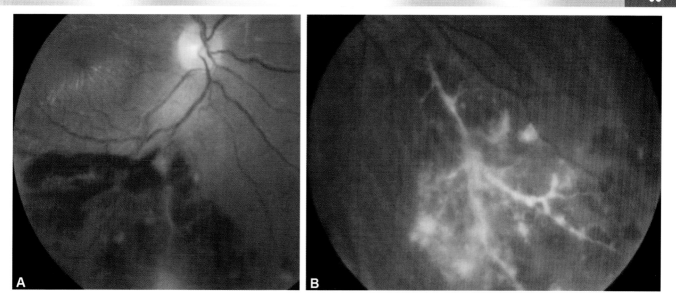

FIGURES 3.20A and B: Sarcoidosis
Unusually severe periphlebitis and macular edema in sarcoid disease of the retina

(Figure 3.20A). Occasionally, when nodular granulomas occur along the retinal vessels, they produce the picture of 'candle-wax droppings' *(Figure 3.20B)*.

Peripheral neovascularization may occur due to ischemia caused by microvascular occlusions. The new vessels tend to cause recurrent vitreous hemorrhage similar to as seen in Eales' disease. Formation of choroidal granulomata is common, in the form of bilateral, multiple, small, pale-yellow elevated lesions, usually most numerous inferiorly. Rarely, papilledema may be seen caused by neurological involvement, even in the absence of other ocular lesions.

4 *Hereditary Diseases*

1. STARGARDT'S MACULAR DYSTROPHY (FUNDUS FLAVIMACULATUS)

Stargardt's disease and fundus maculatus are the different clinical manifestations of genetically the same disease. The former variety is dominated by macular degenerative changes, while appearance of multiple, pale-yellow flecks at the posterior pole is the predominant feature of the other variety. The clinical presentation may be in one or the other form; or both the characteristics may be seen in the same eye. Moreover, within the same family, some members manifest an atrophic macular lesion with or without flecks (Stargardt's disease), while other members can manifest only flecks without an atrophic macular lesion (fundus flavimaculatus).

The disease is most frequently inherited as an autosomal recessive trait. The gene responsible for the transport of retinol to the RPE is the ABCA4 (formerly ABCR) gene. If this gene is defective, transport of retinol cannot take place and the waste remains in the photoreceptor tissue, where the toxic A2E poisons the healthy cells. A2E is a toxic byproduct of vitamin A that is normally released after light exposure during the visual cycle. Dark adaptation is, therefore, affected. As a result, there is deposition of lipofuscins (waste products) within the apical portion of the pigment epithelial cells.

The onset of the disease occurs within the first 10 or 20 years of life when decreased central vision is first noticed. In the early stages of the disease, the patient may have good visual acuity, but may complain of difficulty in reading and seeing in dim light. The disease may be misdiagnosed or not diagnosed in the first few years of the onset because of little evidence being found on fundus examination. Color vision declines as the disease progresses, but patients usually maintain a sufficient amount of color vision.

Stargardt's disease creates central blind spot that increases in size as the disease progresses. Patients learn to turn their eyes in a specific direction to see around the blind spot—'Eccentric viewing'.

Children with Stargardt's disease often complain of difficulty adapting to dark after sunlight exposure.

In more severe cases of vision loss, patients may experience Phantom vision or visual hallucinations (Charles-Bonnet syndrome). This represents a normal attempt by brain to make sense of impaired sensory information. The brain may embellish the image, making it very real just as it does in our dreams.

The degenerative changes at the macula appear as mottling of the macula along with an oval lesion of about 1-1.5 disk diameters in size that has a 'beaten bronze' appearance *(Figure 4.1)*. In some cases, it may be surrounded by a few flecks. Gradually, the lesion becomes more extensive, accompanied with a progressive visual loss.

On the other hand, the form of disease manifesting predominantly in the form of flecks, appears later in life (i.e. in the fourth or fifth decade), and may be discovered by chance in some asymptomatic cases. The characteristic lesions appear as multiple yellow or pale-yellow spots located mostly at the posterior pole. These spots (flecks) may be round, linear, or fishtail (pisciform) in shape. New lesions appear from the periphery as the old lesions resolve leaving behind atrophic areas in the retinal pigment epithelium. With time, all lesions tend to become more extensive and confluent. Visual prognosis largely depends on the frequency and severity of atrophic changes at the macula. In general, it is better than in the category of cases which manifest the disease in the form of macular dystrophy, at an earlier age.

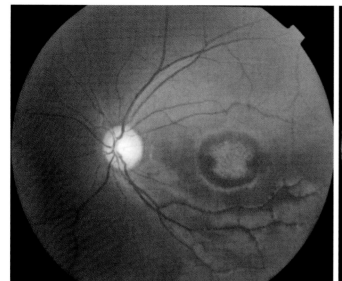

FIGURE 4.1: Stargardt's disease
Degenerative lesion at the macula with
'beaten bronze' appearance

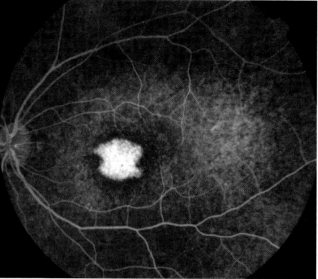

FIGURE 4.2: Stargardt's disease
Angiogram shows hyperfluorescence (window defect)
at the site of lesion

Fundus fluorescein angiography revels hyperfluorescence at the macula, indicative of window defects *(Figure 4.2)*.

Treatment

Currently, there is no effective treatment for Stargardt's disease. Appropriate low vision aids and lighting are two important considerations for helping both the children and adults to function as normally as possible. Genetic manipulation holds some hope for developing new strategies for therapy.

A recent study showed that the formation of A2E is strongly suppressed by treating the ABCR mice with Accutaine (isotretinoin), an inhibitor of rhodopsin regeneration. Similarly, Fenrutinide has shown promising results as another type of A2E suppressor.

2. BESTS' DISEASE (VITELLIFORM DEGENERATION)

Vitelliform degeneration of the macula presents a pleomorphic ophthamoscopic picture. The initial lesion undergoes morphological changes at various stages of its progress. The mode of inheritance is autosomal dominant with incomplete penetrance and variable expressivity. The disorder has been mapped to a genetic defect in chromosome 11. The lesions are bilateral and affect both sexes equally. It is caused by the accumulation of lipofuscin within the cells of retinal pigment epithelium (RPE) and the subepithelial space. A hallmark of the disease is a markedly abnormal electrooculogram (EOG) in all stages of progression as well as in phenotypically normal carriers. Full electroretinogram (ERG) remains normal. Focal ERG concentrated on the macular function may show some abnormality. The abnormal EOG and a normal ERG implicates the retinal pigment epithelium to be the primary seat of malfunction. Family members having normal EOG ratios can, with reasonable assurance, be presumed normal. The role of EOG testing for all immediate family members of affected patients has obvious practical implications for genetic counseling.

Typical bilateral early macular lesions of yellow 'egg-yolk' or 'sunny-side up' appearance are seen ophthalmoscopically *(Figure 4.3),* several years before the symptoms of visual loss are manifest. Most patients are either asymptomatic or show only slight visual loss until between 40 and 50 years of age. The lesions are usually single and located at the macula but occasionally may be multiple. The appearance of the lesion and the onset of visual loss often vary between the two eyes. In general, most people will maintain good vision at least in one eye.

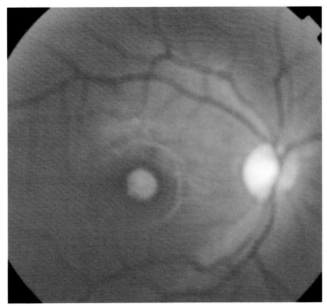

FIGURE 4.3: Best's disease
Vitelliform stage with 'egg-yolk' appearance

Over the years, the lesion exhibits progressive changes in morphology described as different stages:

Stage-1 (previtelliform). Macula looks normal, subtle RPE changes may be seen, and EOG is abnormal.

Stage-2 (vitelliform). There is a well-circumscribed 0.5-5 mm, round, elevated, yellowish lesion centered at the macula (egg-yolk appearance).

*Stage-*3 (pseudo-hypopion). Yellowish material breaks through the RPE and collects subretinally in a cyst with fluid level formation.

Stage-4 (vitelliruptive). It gives scrambled egg appearance due to the breakup of the uniform vitelliform lesion. Visual acuity at this stage may show moderate deterioration.

*Stage-*5 *(atrophic).* The yellowish material disappears with evident RPE atrophy. Vision may be more markedly affected. It may be difficult to differentiate from other forms of macular degeneration.

Stage-6 (chroidal neovascularization). CNV may develop in some eyes following the atrophic stage leading to a whitish subretinal membrane.

Treatment

No treatment exists for vitelliform macular dystrophy. CNV, if present, may be treated with direct laser coagulation. Treatment with intravitreal bevacizumab (Avastin) has also been suggested.

3. CONE DYSTROPHY

Cone dystrophy (*progressive cone dystrophy, cone-rod dystrophy*) is an inherited defect that primarily affects the cone system in both eyes. Lesser degree of rod dysfunction may or may not manifest during the course of disease. The age of onset, rate of progression and ultimate severity of signs and symptoms vary between and even within the affected families. Clinical features can manifest as early as childhood, or as late as middle or late adulthood. The rate of progression and the extent of visual loss are usually worse in early onset cases.

The common mode of inheritance is autosomal dominant. Autosomal recessive and X-linked transmission can also take place. There may be some sporadic cases as well. The gene for cone dystrophy has been mapped to 17p. The X-linked form of cone dystrophy has been mapped to the short arm of the X chromosome.

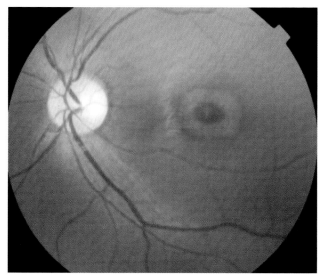

FIGURE 4.4: Cone dystrophy
'Bull's-eye' lesion at the macula with homogeneous, dark central zone surrounding by hypopigmented ring

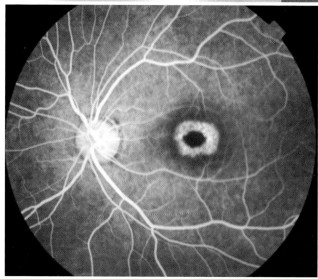

FIGURE 4.5: Cone dystrophy
Angiogram shows a central zone of hypofluorescence surrounded by a ring of hyperfluorescence

The disease presents with the symptoms of photoaversion, day blindness, defective color vision and progressive loss of vision. All these symptoms may precede visible fundus changes. Electroretinography (ERG) and color vision testing helps to reach the diagnosis at this stage of the disease. At first, pigment stippling with diffuse pigment granularity appears at the posterior pole. Later, a characteristic 'Bulls-eye' lesion is seen at the macula that shows a central, homogeneous, dark area surrounded by a hypopigmented zone *(Figure 4.4)*. This is the most common form of lesion observed. It is not possible to predict the prognosis in individual cases but peripheral vision and independent mobility are retained for several years.

Visual field examination reveals a central scotoma. Color vision is grossly defective. The single flash photopic ERG, and the photopic flicker ERG are low or unrecordable.

Fundus fluorescein angiography (FFA) may reveal pigment alterations even before they are visible ophthalmoscopically. Early on, there may be mild, mottled hyperfluorescence. With the appearance of 'Bull's-eye" lesion, FFA shows a discrete, oval area of hyperfluorescence surrounding a hypofluorescent center *(Figure 4.5)*.

Treatment

No means of treatment are available at present. Gene therapy may be available in future.

4. RETINITIS PIGMENTOSA

Retinitis pigmentosa includes a group of inheritable clinical entities with the common factor of progressive loss of photoreceptor and RPE function. With advances in molecular research, it is now known that retinitis pigmentosa is caused by molecular defect in more than 100 different genes. The heterogenicity even extends phenotypically in the sense that patients with the same mutation may have different disease manifestations. Thus, the clinical presentation varies in different patients, as also the different individuals of the same family. Typically, the disease is a diffuse, mostly bilaterally symmetrical retinal dystrophy affecting the rods to a greater degree than the cones. Most patients of retinitis pigmentosa are myopic, and many have keratoconus as well.

Although nearly a quarter of cases occur sporadically, the mode of inheritance may be autosomal dominant (most common), autosomal recessive or uncommonly, X-linked recessive. In a small group of cases, the mode

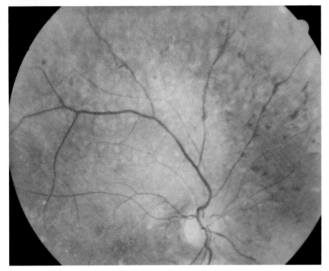

FIGURE 4.6: Retinitis pigmentosa
Pigment spicules in the equatorial region overlying
the retinal veins, at places

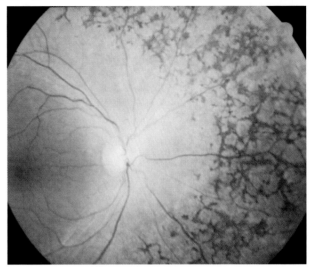

FIGURE 4.7: Retinitis pigmentosa
Coarse, 'bone corpuscle' pigment distributed in the
equatorial zone; macula appears normal

is uncertain. Cases with autosomal dominant transmission have the best prognosis, while the prognosis is worst in cases with X-linked recessive disease.

The disease most commonly presents with night blindness. Nearly three-quarters of the patients develop the symptom by the age of thirty years. The earliest clinical finding consists of arterial narrowing along with fine dust-like intraretinal pigment. Gradually, the pigment becomes coarser assuming bone corpuscle configuration *(Figures 4.6 and 4.7)*. The pigment tends to arrange along the retinal vessels, overlying the veins at places. The lesions involve the mid-periphery of the fundus initially, gradually spreading peripherally as well as centrally. At this stage, the optic disk shows the classical waxy pallor. In the advanced cases, marked tessellation of the fundus is seen and large choroidal vessels may become visible. The macula may show atrophy *(Figures 4.8A and B)*, cellophane maculopathy or cystoid edema which causes a considerable loss of

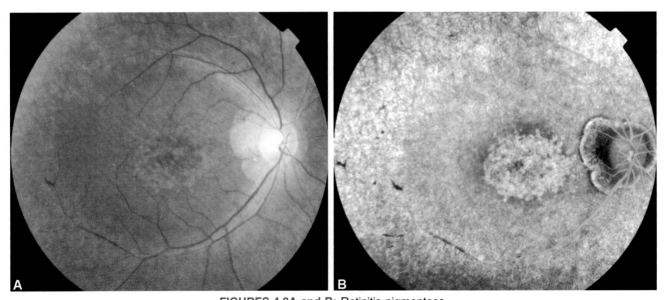

FIGURES 4.8A and B: Retinitis pigmentosa
A. Peripheral pigmentary degeneration associated with macular degeneration
B. Angiogram shows widespread window defects including the macular area, due to RPE atrophy; stray,
small patches of hypofluorescence (blocked fluorescence) are caused by the pigment deposits

central vision in such cases. Posterior subcapsular opacities appear in the lens. Visual fields show a ring scotoma followed by all-round constriction until a small central island is left intact. ERG changes appear in the early stages, even before the fundus changes are obvious. There is reduced amplitude of photopic and scotopic b-wave. Delayed implicit time is present.

Nearly three-quarters of patients maintain good vision and can read despite the tubular (2-5 degrees) visual field. By the age of 50, a considerable number of patients have a very poor vision.

Electroretinography (ERG) is the most critical test for retinitis pigmentosa because it provides an objective measure of rod and cone function across the retina, and is sensitive to even mild photoreceptor impairment. The full field ERG shows a marked reduction of both rod and cone signals, although rod loss usually predominates. The a and b wave are reduced. ERG is abnormal by early childhood but for some very mild and localized disease.

Electrooculography (EOG) findings are always abnormal when ERG is abnormal. Therefore, it is not helpful to the clinician in diagnosing the disease.

Fundus fluorescein angiography (FFA) and optical coherence tomography (OCT) are of little help in the diagnosis of retinitis pigmentosa, but may be useful in confirming the presence and the progress of macular edema, if present.

Examination of visual fields is a very useful measure for ongoing follow-up.

Contrast sensitivity testing shows reduced values, out of proportion to visual acuity, in patients with retinitis pigmentosa.

Genetic subtyping should be of use in devising therapies to target specific genetic subtypes. In addition, subtyping the gene may be helpful in determining the prognosis, and in providing the genetic counseling.

In some cases of retinitis pigmentosa, pigment clumps are invisible ophthalmoscopically, though other features like atrophic disk, narrow vessels and typical ERG changes are present—*retinitis pigmentosa sine pigmento.* Many believe it to be the early cases of the classical disease rather than a separate entity.

Occasionally, the disease has been seen to be present localized to a segment of the retina alone—*Sector retinitis pigmentosa (Figure 4.9).* Such patients show localized fundus changes of constricted retinal vessels, bone-spicule pigmentation within the inner retina around blood vessels and retinal hypopigmentation. These changes are generally bilateral most frequently present in the inferior quadrants.

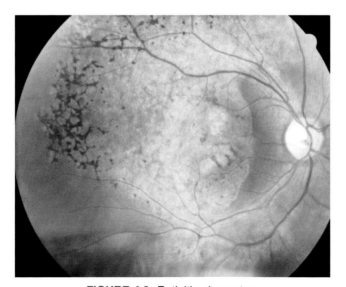

FIGURE 4.9: Retinitis pigmentosa
Disease confined to the upper temporal sector
(sectoral retinitis pigmentosa); macular degeneration is also present

Another variant of the disease is seen in the form of *unilateral retinitis pigmentosa.* When truly present, it manifests with classical fundus changes in one eye, the other eye looking normal. There are minimal or undetectable ERG responses and abnormal EOG ratios in the affected eye and normal ERG and EOG findings in the ophthalmoscopically unaffected eye.

Retinitis pigmentosa is associated with increased prevalence of optic disk drusens, open-angle glaucoma, keratoconus and myopia. It is also associated with a wide variety of systemic disorders which have been described in the form of various syndromes:

1. *Bardet-Biedl (Laurence-Moon) syndrome.* Its five cardinal features include polydactyly or syndactyly, pigmentary retinopathy, obesity, mental retardation and hypogonadism.
2. *Refsum's syndrome.* The main features of this condition include peripheral neuropathy and cerebellar ataxia along with an atypical pigmentary degeneration of retina with night blindness and constriction of visual fields.
3. *Usher's syndrome.* This autosomal recessively inherited syndrome is constituted by a congenital neuro-sensory deafness and retinitis pigmentosa.

Treatment

No specific treatment is available for the treatment of retinitis pigmentosa.

A recent comprehensive epidemiologic study concluded that high doses of vitamin A (15,000 units per day) in the form of vitamn A palmitate, slow the progress of retinitis pigmentosa by about 20% per year. Supplements of beta carotenes, the natural precursors of vitamin A, are not a predictable source of the vitamin as each person breaks down the beta carotenes differently. The dose of vitamin A needs adjustments in cases with liver disease and in cases with pre-existing high levels of vitamin A.

In this study, the disease appeared to progress faster on a daily, 400 iu of vitamin E supplementation than those taking a trace amount of the vitamin.

Docosahexaeonic acid (DHA) administration has been reported to reduce ERG changes. However, a recent study compared DHA & vitamin A to vitamin A alone in patients of retinitis pigmentosa, for 4 years. Benefit of DHA was not seen.

Studies have demonstrated improvement of visual acuity with oral acetazolamide in eyes which had retinitis pigmentosa with macular edema.

Lucin and Zeaxanthin are thought to protect the macula from oxidative damage, and oral supplementation has been seen to increase the macular pigment. Ongoing study is in progress to study its effect in cases of wet ARMD.

Ciliary Neurotrophic Factor (CNF) has been observed to slow down retinal degeneration in a number of animal models. Phase II clinical trials are underway, using an encapsulated form of RPE-cell producing CNF, placed surgically in to the eye. Phase I trials have been encouraging.

Transplantation of patches of retinal or RPE tissue; RPE cell transplantation in the subretinal space, and stem cell transplants are being studied in animal models. No current investigational protocol exists in humanns for this type of investigation.

Retinal prosthesis or phototransducing chip placed on the retinal surface in order to stimulate healthy ganglion cells, has been investigated for several years. Other models have also been designed. This technology remains investigational, and currently no prosthesis is available for clinical use.

Gene therapy is under investigation with the hope to replace the defective protein by using DNA vector.

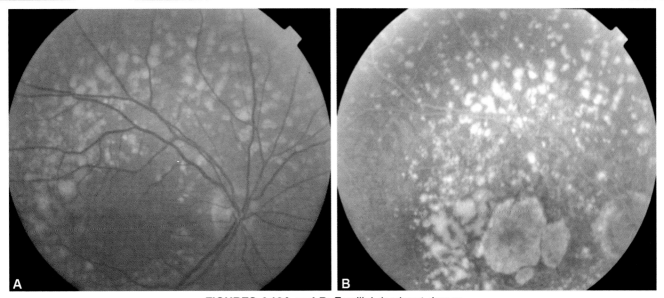

FIGURES 4.10A and B: Familial dominant drusen
A. Large, confluent, soft drusen in a 55-year-old female with similar lesions amongst the siblings
B. Beside the spots of hyperfluorescence over the drusen, a large window defect is present over the macula caused by the atrophy of overlying RPE—Dry ARMD

5. FAMILIAL DOMINANT DRUSEN

It is inherited as an autosomal dominant trait with variable penetrance and expressivity. The underlying factor is presumed to be at the level of pigment epithelium because of an inborn error in the metabolism of these cells.

Familial drusen of the Bruch's membrane generally appear first between the ages of 20 and 30 years and tend to increase in size after 40 years. Drusen present nasal to the optic disk are supposed to provide a diagnostic criterion for its being of familial nature. During the fifth or sixth decade of life, the drusen become increasingly more confluent, visual acuity may be affected as atrophic changes in the retinal pigment epithelium and the overlying sensory retina become more extensive *(Figures 4.10A and B)*. Choroidal neovascularization is sometimes seen in elderly individuals.

6. CENTRAL AREOLAR CHOROIDAL SCLEROSIS (SYN. CENTRAL AREOLAR CHOROIDAL DYSTROPHY)

It is a rare, bilateral disorder often challenging to diagnose because of the many chorioretinal conditions with similar funduscopic findings. It is characterized by a circumscribed area of atrophy with disappearance of pigment epithelium, choriocapillaries and the photoreceptors in the macular area, traversed by choroidal vessels *(Figures 4.11A and B)*. Characteristically, there is a gradual loss of vision manifesting in the fifth decade. Central scotoma is present. Autosomal dominant, autosomal recessive and sporadic cases have been reported. Fundus examination shows bilateral areas of atrophy at the macula of 1-3 disk diameters in size. Large choroidal vessels are visible at the base of the lesions. Some amount of irregular pigmentation may be present. The lesions are progressive and carry poor visual prognosis.

Treatment

No effective treatment is known for central areolar choroidal sclerosis.

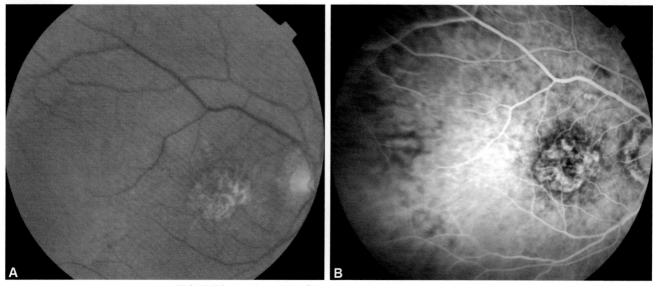

FIGURES 4.11A and B: Central areolar choroidal sclerosis
A. Circumscribed patch of atrophy of the RPE and choriocapillaries located at the macula
B. Angiogram shows transmitted fluorescence from the large choroidal vessels

Chapter 5

Optic Nerve Disorders

1. MYELINATED NERVE FIBERS

A commonly seen asymptomatic condition, it is present unilaterally, or on occasions, bilaterally. It represents a developmental anomaly that is thought to be due to the presence of ectopic oligodendrocyte-like cells in the retina. Feather-like white patch radiating from the disk characterizes it *(Figure 5.1)*. Other patterns may also be present such as an isolated patch that is not continuous with the optic nerve head, peripapillary myelination or extensive myelination starting at the disk and extending towards the periphery *(Figures 5.2 and 5.3)*. The incidence of myelinated nerve fibers has been reported from 0.57 to 0.98%. The myelinated patches may or may not obscure the retinal blood vessels.

Generally believed to be benign, there are several reports of its association with unilateral high myopia and amblyopia, especially in eyes with widespread myelination. Association of optic disk dysplasia and pseudo-macular hole has also been reported. In another study, it was observed that neuroretinal rim and rim-to-disk area ratio was significantly less than that of fellow eyes with no myelination. This may be taken into consideration when monitoring glaucoma suspects with peripapillary myelinated nerve fibers.

Disappearance of the existing myelinated fibers is indicative of optic atrophy.

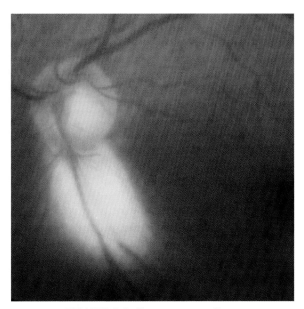

FIGURE 5.1: Opaque nerve fibers
Feather-like, white patch radiating from the optic disk

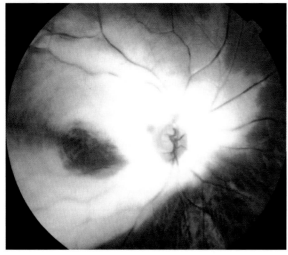

FIGURE 5.2: Opaque nerve fibers
Extensive myelination surrounding the entire
circumference of the optic disk, and radiating
towards the periphery

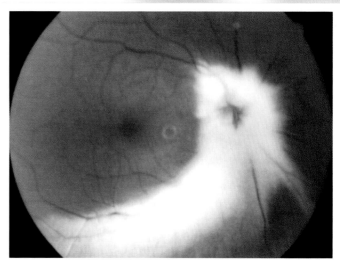

FIGURE 5.3: Opaque nerve fibers
Extensive myelination

2. OPTIC DISK COLOBOMA

A coloboma of the optic disk is the result of defective closure of the embryonic ventral fissure. In keeping with the location of the embryonic fissure, the typical coloboma is located inferiorly and slightly nasally. It may vary from a focal, small excavation to a widespread defect associated with the coloboma of choroid and the ciliary body *(Figure 5.4)*. In either case, poor vision is present. Retinal detachment of non-rhegmatogenous type is frequently seen.

The retinochoroidal coloboma that involves the optic disk is usually bilateral. It is characterized by a strikingly white ectatic zone in the inferior fundus that extends into and distorts the optic disk. Within the colobomatous optic disk, the nerve is usually atrophic. Scattered areas of pigmentation may be present because of hyperplasia of the RPE.

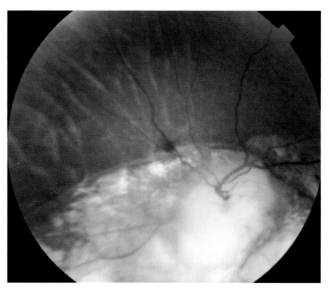

FIGURE 5.4: Coloboma of optic disk
Coloboma of the disk as a component of a large coloboma involving the choroid, and ciliary body

If the coloboma affects the optic nerve alone, the optic disk becomes enlarged and deeply cupped. Persistent hyaloid remnants are often present. The radial arrangement of the vessels emerging from the edge of the disk (like spokes of a wheel) is referred to as *'morning glory syndrome'* .

3. OPTIC DISK PIT

Congenital optic disk pits appear as unilateral (85%), small craters or holes most commonly in the infer-temporal part of the optic disk. The size of the pit may vary from one-third to half of the optic disk size, has steep walls, and its base is usually pigmented giving it a gray appearance *(Figure 5.5).* The optic disk looks larger than the normal, in eyes with optic pits. Nearly half of the eyes with optic disk pit have cilioretinal arteries. Such eyes are most vulnerable to the development of normal tension glaucoma. Unlike the colobomata, no embryogenic explanation is available for this anomaly.

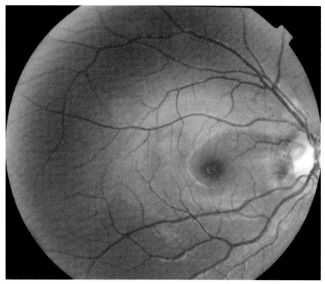

FIGURE 5.5: Optic disk pit
Pigmented pit in the upper temporal part of the optic disk

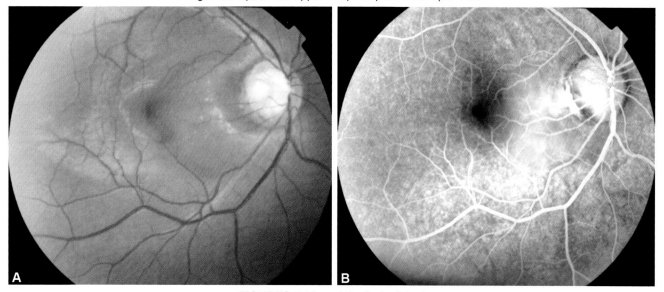

FIGURES 5.6A and B: Optic disk pit
A. Scantily pigmented pit, complicated with detachment of the sensory retina over the macula
B. Unlike in CSR, the sensory detachment of the macular retina associated with optic disk pit does not reveal any evidence of dye leakage on fluorescein angiography

Although optic pits may cause an enlargement of blind spot and an arcuate, paracentral, or cecocentral scotoma, most of the patients are asymptomatic and are unaware of the disease unless associated with the complication of the development of detachment of sensory retina at the macula *(Figures 5.6A and B)*. Nearly half of the cases have this complication of serous maculopathy. A careful assessment of the optic disk to exclude the presence of optic disk pit is important to differentiate it from the clinical entity of central serous retinopathy. Of greater significance, however, is the fact that spontaneous improvement of serous maculopathy seldom occurs in eyes with optic disk pit, leading to a very poor visual prognosis owing to the formation of a macular cyst or a hole.

The question of whether the subretinal fluid is derived from vitreous humor, cerebrospinal fluid, or possibly the result of macular traction is debatable. New findings strongly suggest that serous macular detachments secondary to optic pits develop due to pre-existing schisis like lesions which connect the macula with the optic disk. Fluid, predominately from the outer plexiform layer of the retina, enters an already edematous retina through the optic pit via the retinal stroma, producing macular detachment.

Treatment

Prophylactic laser coagulation, therapeutic laser coagulation after the maculopathy has developed, oral steroids, and vitrectomy have been tried. The current trend is to perform laser coagulation following the onset of serous maculopathy.

4. OPTIC DISK DRUSEN

Optic disk drusen are composed of hyaline-like material within the substance of the optic nerve head. They are seen clinically in 1% population, but nearly three times more commonly in individuals with a family history of optic disk drusen. In nearly three-quarters of cases, both eyes are involved. Suspectedly, the mode of inheritance is of an autosomal dominant pattern with incomplete penetrance, and associated with inherited dysplasia of the optic disk and its blood supply. Certain conditions, such as retinitis pigmentosa, angioid streaks, and Usher's syndrome may be associated with optic disk drusen. The drusen are believed to be the result of abnormal axoplasmic metabolism followed by axonal degradation, mitochondrial calcification and mucoprotein deposition.

In children, the drusen are generally buried and undetectable by funduscopy, although a mild-to-moderate elevation of the optic disk may be present. Ultrasonography is of help to reach the diagnosis. With age, overlying axons become atrophied and the drusen become exposed and more visible *(Figures 5.7A and B)*. The drusen may be discrete or multi-globular with ill-defined margins. The optic disk appears waxy, white-yellow, and swollen (*pseudopapilledema*). Fundus fluorescein angiography is helpful in distinguishing it from true papilledema.

Optic disk drusen can compress and eventually compromise the vasculature and the optic nerve fibers. Central vision is compromised in the eventuality of the development of CNV. The optic disk damage is progressive and insidious. Eventually, nearly three-fourths of the patients develop field defects. There can be nasal step defects, enlarged blind spots, arcuate scotoma, sectoral field loss, and altitudinal defects. Rarely, choroidal neovascularization (CNV) may develop as the juxtapapillary fibers get disrupted. Visual impairment may be caused because of peripapillary choroidal neovascularization. Development of anterior ischemic optic neuropathy (AION) is a potential complication.

Treatment

There is no widely accepted treatment for optic disk drusen. Some clinicians recommend prescribing local drops that reduce intraocular pressure, to relieve mechanical stress on fibers of the optic disk. Peripapillary CNV that may be rarely seen is treated with laser coagulation, photodynamic therapy, or other evolving therapies.

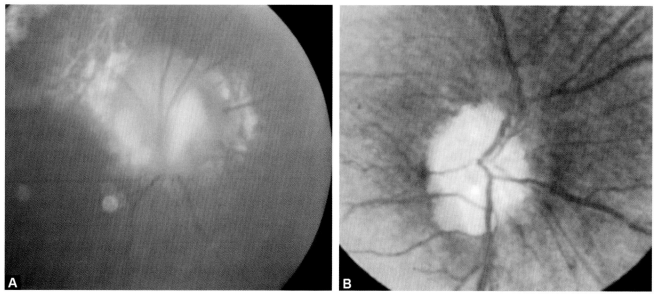

FIGURES 5.7A and B: Optic disk drusen
With exposure of the drusen, optic disk looks swollen (pseudopapilledema)

Clinical monitoring in the follow-up is supplemented with optic coherence tomography (OCT) to evaluate the nerve fiber layer thickness.

5. PAPILLEDEMA

Papilledema is defined as swelling of the optic nerve head secondary to raised intracranial pressure. The term 'disk swelling' is employed for edema of the optic disk caused by any other factor than the raised intracranial pressure. It is mostly bilateral, though may be asymmetrical. Various types of intracranial tumors (space-occupying lesions) provide the most common cause for the increase in the intracranial pressure. Some of the other common causes include benign intracranial hypertension, diffuse cerebral edema and severe hypertension. Appearance of papilledema is the direct result of raised intracranial pressure that is transmitted along the common meningeal sheaths of the brain and optic nerves producing engorged, swollen disk. The swelling results primarily because of axoplasmic stasis, or slowed cellular conduction along the nerve. Consequently, intracellular fluids and metabolic byproducts accumulate and are eventually regurgitated at the level of optic nerve head.

Early papilledema *(Figure 5.8)* is mostly devoid of visual symptoms, and manifests in the form of hyperemia of the disk, blurring of the disk margins (nasal margins are the first to be involved), and loss of spontaneous venous pulsations, if known to be present earlier.

In a case of well-established papilledema, the patient may complain of episodes of transient obscuring of vision, lasting for a few seconds. General symptoms of headache, nausea, and vomiting are usually present. Headache typically is worse on awakening and on coughing. Diplopia may be present if the sixth cranial nerve is compromised. Visual acuity may be normal or reduced.

The optic disk shows *(Figures 5.9 and 5.10)* severe hyperemia along with a variable degree of elevation. There is engorgement of retinal veins with flame-shaped hemorrhages in the peripapillary zone. Cotton-wool spots are often present. Hard exudates are seen radiating from the macula in the shape of an incomplete star with its temporal part missing *(macular fan)*. In the case of a long-standing papilledema, visual acuity is impaired significantly. The optic disk shows pallor, indistinct margins, with fewer crossing blood vessels. This appearance is referred to as *'secondary post-neuritic optic atrophy'*.

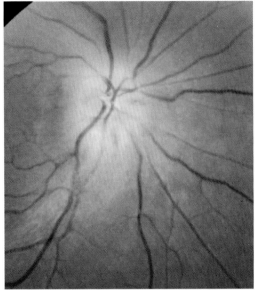

FIGURE 5.8: Papilledema
Moderate degree of papilledema shows
hyperemic optic disk with hazy margins, filled up
physiological cup, dilated retinal veins, and a few
hemorrhages over and around the disk

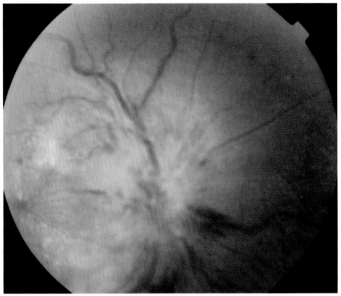

FIGURE 5.9: Papilledema
Severe degree of papilledema with obvious swelling
grossly dilated retinal veins, multiple retinal
hemorrhages, and a few cotton-wool spots

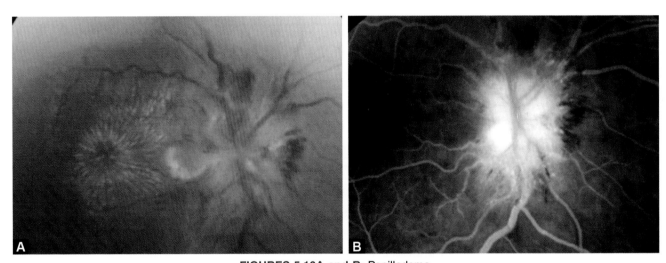

FIGURES 5.10A and B: Papilledema
A. Severe papilledema with macular star formation
B. Angiogram shows hyperfluorescence over and around the optic disk;
areas of blocked fluorescence caused by retinal hemorrhages

Visual field examination shows enlargement of blind spot in the acute stage, and peripheral constriction of field in longstanding cases. In cases with extreme edema of the disk, a pseudobitemporal hemianopsia may be elicited. CT scan and MRI of skull is performed to look for the underlying causative factor. Occasionally, OCT may be required to differentiate it from buried drusen of the optic disk (pseudopapilledema). Fluorescein angiography is indicated to confirm the diagnosis, in doubtful cases.

Treatment

The treatment is directed to manage the causative factor. Diuretics like acetazolamide may be administered in selected cases, especially in cases of benign intracranial hypertension (BIH). Surgical decompression of the optic nerve sheath, by creating a small fenestration site within the intraorbital portion of the optic nerve, may be performed to relieve symptoms in medically controlled cases of BIH. The decompression procedure is complex and fails to work in nearly one-third cases.

6. OPTIC NEURITIS

Inflammations of the optic nerve manifest in the following clinical forms:

(i) *Retrobulbar neuritis.* In this condition the inflammation is confined to the post-laminar part of the optic nerve. The optic nerve head is spared, and appears normal. It is the most common type of manifestation in adults and is frequently associated with multiple sclerosis.

(ii) *Papillitis.* In this condition the optic nerve head is affected in the form of hyperemia and edema *(Figures 5.11A and B).* Occasionally, a few flame-shaped hemorrhages may be present around the optic disk. A few vitreous cells are present in the posterior part. It is seen more frequently in children.

(iii) *Neuroretinitis.* It is characterized by papillitis accompanied by collection of hard exudates in a star fashion around the macula. The hard exudates usually appear a few days after the disk swelling, and tend to become more prominent when the optic disk edema is resolving *(Figure 5.12).* At times, there may be peripapillary edema and a sensory detachment of the macula. It is a self-limiting condition that resolves within 6-12 months. No association with multiple sclerosis has been noted.

Adult optic neuritis. Optic neuritis is a demyelinating inflammation of the optic nerve. Many cases occur in association with multiple sclerosis (MS), but isolated cases occur frequently. Optic neuritis is frequently the first manifestation in cases of MS. Long-term follow up suggests that 75% of females with optic neuritis manifest other lesions of MS, in due course of time. Some infective processes involving the orbits or paranasal sinuses can also cause optic neuritis, or it may develop during the course of a viral illness. Optic neuritis is believed to be an autoimmune reaction resulting in demyelinating inflammation.

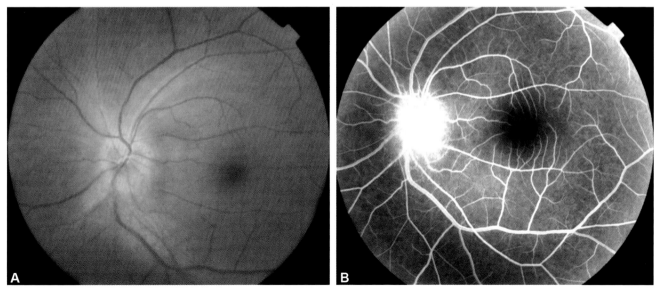

FIGURES 5.11A and B: Papillitis
A. Hyperemia and hazy margins of the optic nerve head; dilated veins
B. Angiogram shows hyperfluorescence over and around the optic disk

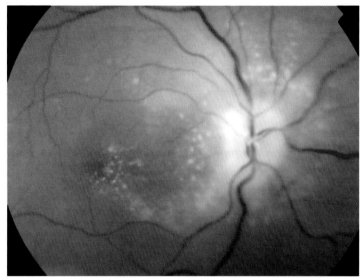

FIGURE 5.12: Neuroretinitis
Resolving swelling of the optic disk with hard exudates on and around the macula

Typically, patients with the first time attack are young healthy adults aged 20-45 years. It is not uncommon to see a bilateral involvement in children, as well.

During the attack, the patients experience rapidly developing impairment of vision in one eye, or less commonly in both eyes. Change in color perception (Dyschromatopsia) is a prominent complaint. Visual symptoms are usually accompanied, or preceded, by retrobulbar pain that is exaggerated on ocular movements. There may be a previous history of such attacks. Patients associated with MS are likely to have recurrences.

Pupillary light reaction is decreased in the affected eye, and a relative afferent pupillary defect (RAPD) can be elicited. Reduction of visual acuity may be from mild-to-complete loss of vision. Almost all patients with visual loss have reduced contrast sensitivity, and defective color vision. Visual fields typically, show a central or cecocentral scotoma. However, according to Optic Neuritis Treatment Trial (ONTT), altitudinal field defects, arcuate defects, and nasal steps are more common than a central or cecocentral scotoma. The fundus may look normal as nearly 2/3 cases have the inflammation limited to the retrobulbar portion of the optic nerve (retrobulbar neuritis). With time, these cases show pallor of the optic disk. The remaining 1/3 cases have swollen disks (papillitis). The disk edema is often diffuse.

Recovery takes place in 4-6 weeks or occasionally, longer. In most cases, the visual acuity recovers to near normal level but the defective color vision, impaired contrast sensitivity and RAPD may persist along with optic atrophy especially in eyes with recurrences.

Magnetic Resonance Imaging (MRI) is a sensitive and specific tool in the assessment of inflammatory changes in the optic nerve, and helps to rule out structural lesions. In addition, MRI may be of help in predicting future development of MS in patients presenting with first time attack of optic neuritis; 10-20% of these patients may have clinically silent demyelinating lesions elsewhere in the brain.

Visually Evoked Responses (VEPs) often show a loss of P100 response in the acute phase. The abnormal response may be seen, even in the presence of normal MRI findings. Moreover, in a suspected case of MS without visual symptoms, abnormal response is suggestive of subclinical involvement of optic nerve.

Treatment

Intravenous steroids (methyl-prednisolone-250 mg, qid for three days) along with a tapering dose of oral steroids, shorten the course of the disease, though it does not influence the final visual outcome. Admission to the hospital is advisable while undertaking intravenous therapy, in view of the risk of serious side effects of this treatment. The ONTT showed strong evidence against the use of oral steroids in isolation, in the treatment of optic neuritis because it may increase the risk of recurrence of optic neuritis.

Childhood Optic Neuritis

In children, most cases of optic neuritis are due to an immune-mediated process. These cases are associated with a viral or other infection or with immunization. Less commonly, optic neuritis may be the first manifestation of multiple sclerosis, or part of a more diffuse demyelinating disorder, such as acute disseminated encephalomyelitis or Devick's dieases. Optic neuritis may result, also from the diseases of the neighboring paranasal sinuses and orbital structures. Infective and infiltrative inflammations of the meninges and brain are one of the common causes of inflammation of the optic nerve in this country.

Clinical manifestations of the childhood neuritis differ in many respects, from those seen in the adult form of the disease. Childhood neuritis is more often bilateral. Papillitis is more common than retrobulbar neuritis seen in the adult variety. It is commonly associated with headache rather than pain around the eye on ocular movements. It follows infections (usually viral) or immunization rather than being idiopathic. There is a lower probability of recurrent demyelinating episodes and diagnosis of multiple sclerosis. Tubercular meningitis is a common cause of optic neuritis in children in this country.

Treatment

Chances of spontaneous recovery of visual acuity are good but for infiltrative inflammations following tuber meningitis. However, some clinicians believe that there is a greater prevalence of steroid responsive and steroid-dependent cases amongst children and recommend treating all the patients with high doses of corticosteroids. According to another opinion, smaller doses are required. In the absence of a related prospective study, no consensus exists for intravenous use of steroids.

7. OPTIC ATROPHY

It is a condition that results as a consequence of a variety of local and systemic disorders. It presents in the form of pallor of the optic disk along with a decrease/absence of small vessels on its surface. According to the ophthalmoscopic picture, it is termed as *primary, secondary (postneuritic), consecutive,* or *glaucomatous* optic atrophy.

Primary optic atrophy refers to the appearance of the optic disk *(Figure 5.13)* where its color is chalky-white, the margins are sharp and well defined, and the physiological cup is enlarged but shallow *(saucer-shaped cup).* The retinal vessels have reduced caliber. It is the result of the lesions of the optic nerve not associated with swelling of the optic nerve head.

Secondary optic atrophy (Figure 5.14) is characterized by the pallor of the optic disk that is not as marked as in the case of primary optic atrophy, and is somewhat dirty white rather than chalky white. The margins of the optic disk are blurred, the optic cup is filled up, and the retinal veins may exhibit tortuosity with or without sheathing in the peripapillary zone. This is the result of optic nerve lesions which are associated with the swelling of the optic nerve head, such as papillitis and papilledema.

Consecutive optic atrophy results as a consequence of degeneration of the retinal neurons, best exemplified by retinitis pigmentosa and central retinal artery occlusion *(Figure 5.15).* Characteristically, the color of the optic disk is waxy pale. The retinal vessels show considerable narrowing.

Glaucomatous optic atrophy results from a diffuse loss of nerve fibers at the optic disk. This loss may be localized [causing notching of the disk *(Figure 5.16)*], or generalized [causing concentric enlargement *[Figure 5.17)*] of the optic disk cup. As the damage progresses, the temporal followed by the nasal disk becomes atrophic. Eventually, all neural tissue at the disk is destroyed and the optic nerve head appears white and deeply excavated *(Figures 5.16 and 5.17).* The deep cup has overhanging margins causing an apparent loss in the continuity of retinal vessels as they travel from the center to the rim of the disk.

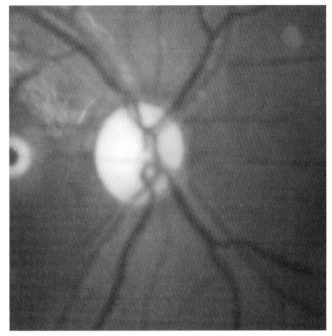

FIGURE 5.13: Optic atrophy
Primary optic atrophy with clear margins and chalky white
color of the optic disk; shallow, saucer-shaped cupping

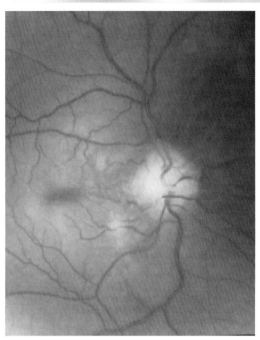

FIGURE 5.14: Optic atrophy
Secondary (postneuritic) optic atrophy with dirty
white color, blurred margins, and filled up cup of
the optic disk; dilated retinal veins

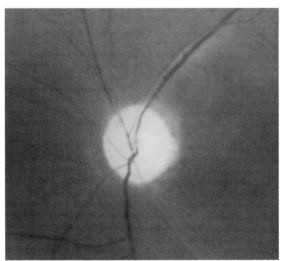

FIGURE 5.15: Optic atrophy
Consecutive optic atrophy with waxy-pale color
and clear margins; narrow retinal vessels
especially the arteries

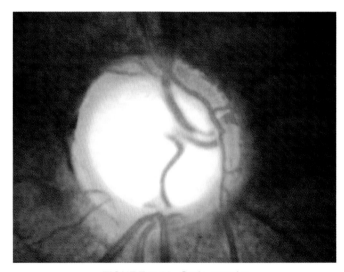

FIGURE 5.16: Optic atrophy
Glaucomatous optic atrophy with deep and enlarged cup
extending to the margins of the optic disk; apparent
discontinuity of blood vessels at the margins

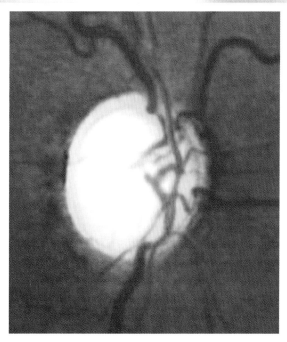

FIGURE 5.17: Optic atrophy
Glaucomatous optic atrophy with enlarged cup

8. AVULSION OF OPTIC DISK

It results from a blunt trauma to the eyeball. The force of impact causes a concussion effect on the globe leading to tearing of the optic nerve fibers at the optic canal. No structure of the optic nerve head is visible. It is accompanied by a variable amount of retinal and vitreous hemorrhage *(Figure 5.18)*. It causes a complete loss of vision.

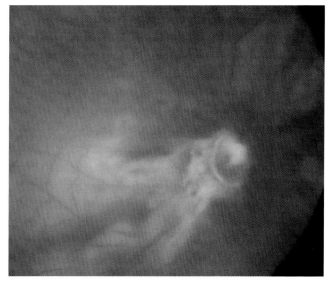

FIGURE 5.18: Avulsion of optic disk
Non-visibility of optic nerve structures; extensive retinal hemorrhages

Tumors

1. CHOROIDAL NEVUS

Choroidal nevi, especially small ones, are of common occurrence. Estimated prevalence of nevi has been reported to be 5-10% in White population. These are perhaps, present at birth and increase in size at puberty. Histologically, nevi are benign neoplasms of the melanocytes located in the outer layers of choroid. The melanocytes are normal in form and function.

A choroidal nevus appears as a flat or minimally raised, slate gray or gray black, round or oval patch, beneath the retina *(Figure 6.1)*. In nearly 10% cases, nevi may be non-pigmented. The size of the lesion is less than 5 mm in diameter and 1 mm in thickness. The margins are typically indistinct. Drusen may be seen overlying the nevus. There is low risk of malignant change.

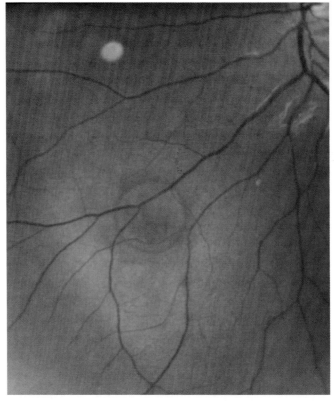

FIGURE 6.1: Choroidal nevus
Solitary, grayish black, round patch beneath the retina

Mostly asymptomatic, nevi have the potential for compromising the visual functions, especially if they are located in the macular area. Thicker nevi may compress the overlying choriocapillaries causing obstruction to the blood supply to retinal pigment epithelium (RPE) and outer segments of photoreceptors, resulting in degeneration of the RPE and photoreceptors. Another serious complication observed is the occurrence of serous detachment of RPE and retina, and choroidal vascularization (CNV). A recent review of more than 3,000 cases of choroidal nevi showed that an estimated risk for visual loss over a period of 15 years was 2% in patients with extrafoveal nevi, but 26% for patients with subfoveal nevi. Choroidal nevi are frequently associated with field defects that are asymptomatic, especially in cases where the nevi are located in the periphery.

Studies suggest that some choroidal melanomas may evolve from malignant transformation within pre-existing nevi. However, the rate of malignant transformation is very low. Estimates of annual rate of transformation vary from one in 4,800 to 8,800. Clinically, risk factors or a possible malignant transformation include tumor thickness of more than 2 mm, documented growth of the tumor, absence of drusen, presence of subretinal fluid, visual symptoms, orange pigment, and posterior margin of the tumor touching the optic disk.

Imaging techniques are helpful in evaluating the potential for malignancy. The presence of internal quite zone on ultrasonography (USG), and hot spots on fundus fluorescein angiography (FFA) have been shown to be predictive of malignancy. Optical coherence tomography (OCT) may be of value in differentiating between active subretinal fluid where the retina overlying the lesion is elevated but otherwise normal in appearance, and chronic changes such as retinal thinning, or intraretinal cysts.

Treatment

No treatment is needed for choroidal nevi. Regular monitoring, along with photographic records, is necessary to detect any possible transformation to malignancy. Imaging procedures are conducted in case of suspicion. In general, nevi of up to 2 mm in size are considered harmless and need yearly check along with photographic documentation, and, if suspicious, B-Scan may be obtained. Nevi of 2-5 mm size are more suspicious, and need 6-monthly observation. In case of suspicion, FFA may be performed. Nevi greater than 5 mm are considered to be melanomas unless proved otherwise.

2. CONGENITAL HYPERTROPHY OF THE RETINAL PIGMENT EPITHELIUM (CHRPE)

It is a peculiar congenital condition of the retinal pigment epithelium (RPE), presenting with characteristic ophthalmoscopic picture. It is asymptomatic and prevalent in 1% of population. It is a benign condition where the pigmentary lesions are unilateral or sometimes, bilateral, solitary or multifocal. The multiple lesions are variably sized, oval or round in shape with sharply demarcated borders. The multiple lesions are located in a pattern *(Figure 6.2)* simulating animals' footprints *(bear-track pigmentation)*. Although CHRPE lesion is usually benign and non-progressive, it can give rise to malignant tumor, on rare occasions.

Bilateral, multiple lesions of CHRPE have been frequently associated with familial adenoid polyposis-FAP (Gardener's disease), an autosomal dominant disease with 100% chance of acquiring malignancy. It has been suggested that CHRPE is an essential extra-colonic abnormality in FAP, both the conditions developing from the same gene. Amongst the offspring of FAP patients, children and young adults having CHRPE lesions are considered to be at risk for FAP. Ocular examination is, therefore, valuable for detecting carriers of the gene for FAP before they develop symptoms.

Currently, however, the CHRPE lesions are considered to constitute two distinct groups. The multifocal, so-called bear track form of CHRPE is often confined to a specific area within the fundus, is usually unilateral, the lesions varying from very small to many disk diameter size. The patches of CHRPE that are associated with FAP are described as atypical, being oval or even fishtail like in shape, bilateral, more isolated in position rather than grouped together, and variable in size up to approximately one DD. Bilateral lesions with a depigmented halo are the hallmarks of CHRPE associated with FAP.

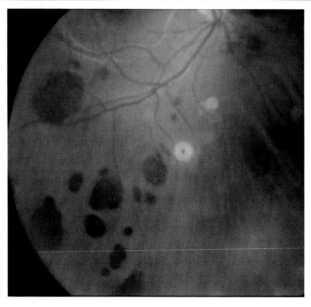

FIGURE 6.2: CHRPE
Multiple, grayish black patches of varying shapes and sizes, located in a pattern
simulating animals' footprints–bear track pigmentation

Treatment

Periodic examination and serial photography is all that is required for the lesions considered typical and not associated with FAP. Consultation with the gastroenterologist is necessary for all lesions suspected to be associated with familial adenoid polyposis.

3. CAPILLARY HEMANGIOMA

Capillary hemangiomas of the retina most likely, represent a vascular hamartoma. These are rare, benign tumors of the retina manifesting in two variations in the form of peripheral retinal hemangioma, and less frequently, the capillary hemangioma of the optic nerve head and/or juxtapapillary retina. Either variant can be associated with von Hippel-Lindau disease. Hereditary and non-hereditary forms are seen.

Retinal capillary hemangiomas usually manifest in the second or third decade of life affecting both sexes with equal frequency. Initially, the lesions may be asymptomatic and discovered on a routine ophthalmic examination. Early symptoms include a decrease in visual acuity and visual field loss. When untreated, the tumor enlarges in size and causes subretinal and retinal exudation *(Figures 6.3A and B)*, eventually culminating in exudative retinal detachment.

Peripheral retinal hemangioma of the retina is often multifocal and bilateral. The peripheral tumors are very small to begin with, resembling a telangiectatic vessel or microaneurysm without any feeder vessel. Gradually, they assume a characteristic appearance of a reddish or gray nodule in the peripheral retina and is supplied by enlarge, tortuous feeder vessel. Fundus fluorescein angiography is helpful in establishing the diagnosis and locating all the lesions.

The capillary hemangioma of the optic nerve head is well circumscribed and easily diagnosed on ophthalmoscopy *(Figures 6.4A and B)*. Blanching of the tumor may be elicited on applying pressure to the globe during examination.

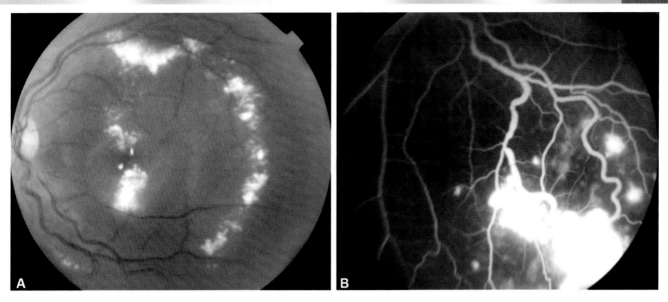

FIGURES 6.3A and B: Capillary hemangioma
A. Subretinal exudation in capillary hemangioma of retina
B. Hyperfluorescent angiomas with feeder vessels

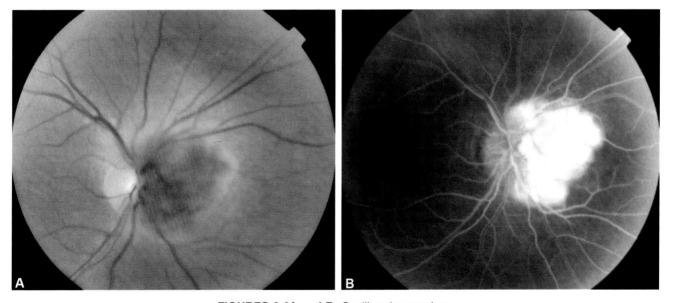

FIGURES 6.4A and B: Capillary hemangioma
A. Well-circumscribed hemangiomatous mass on the optic disk
B. Hyperfluorescence from the tumor

Treatment

Eyes with untreated angiomas have a poor prognosis because of the associated macular exudation and exudative retinal detachment. Early treatment of peripheral capillary hemangiomas with laser or xenon photocoagulation is advocated.

4. ASTROCYTOMA

Astrocytoma of the retina or the optic nerve is a rare, benign tumor that does not threaten the visual functions. It may be seen as of an isolated occurrence but, most frequently, it represents a component of tuberous sclerosis (Bournville's disease). Tuberous sclerosis is an autosomal dominant disease caused by mutations in either TSC1 or TSC2, with loss of hamartin or tuberin functions. It is characterized by enhanced proliferation of neural and astrocyte precursors. The disease manifests with neurologic, cutaneous, visceral, and retinal lesions.

Optic disk elevation in tuberous sclerosis is usually attributable to an astrocytic hamartoma on the surface of the optic disk. The early lesion appears as a focal elevated mass of whitish, gray, or yellowish tissue on the surface of optic disk, masking the underlying retinal vessels in the neighborhood *(Figures 6.5A and B)*. These phakomas generally do not grow, and gradually calcify. The calcified lesion appears as a raised tumor with a 'mulberry-like' appearance that is also seen in some cases of optic disk drusen.

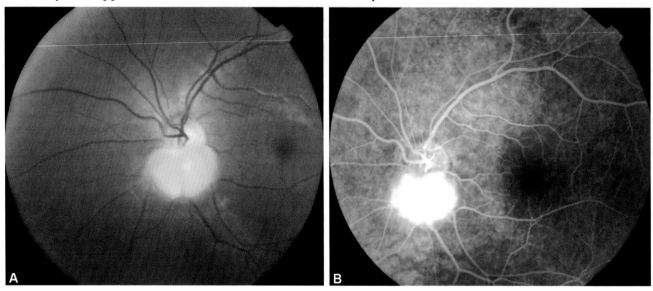

FIGURES 6.5A and B: Astrocytoma of optic disk
A. Elevated pale-pink mass on the optic disk, masking the underlying vessels
B. Hyperfluorescence from the tumor

There are reports describing a progressive increase in the size of the optic disk, and gradual expansion of the lesion into the peripapillary subretinal space. Such lesions, perhaps, represent occasional cases of low-grade intrapapillary tumors.

5. MELANOCYTOMA

Although it can be present in any part of the uveal tract, optic nerve head is the most common site for the tumor. It is more frequently seen in dark skinned people.

Most tumors are asymptomatic and discovered on a routine examination. Evidence of optic nerve dysfunction may be seen occasionally in deep seated tumors. It appears as a black and flat patch with feathery margins, usually located in the inferior part of optic disk *(Figure 6.6)*. It remains stable or may grow slowly, rarely changing to malignant melanoma.

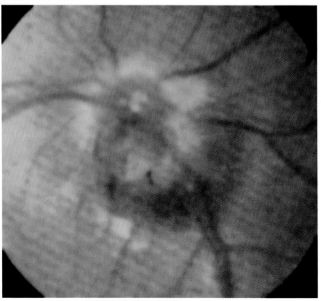

FIGURE 6.6: Melanocytoma
Black, flat patch over the lower part of optic disk

Retinal Detachment

INTRODUCTION

Next to central retinal artery occlusion and perforating or chemical trauma to the eye, retinal detachment is one of the most time-critical eye emergencies. Retinal detachment is a condition where the sensory layers of the retina are separated from the retinal pigment epithelium (RPE) by any of the following mechanisms:

- Holes, tears, or breaks in the retina allowing fluid from the vitreous cavity to seep in between the sensory layers of retina and RPE (*rhegmatogenous retinal detachment*).
- Traction from membranes of inflammatory or vascular origin (such as in Eales' disease, proliferative diabetic retinopathy etc.) pulling the retina forward *(Figure 7.1)*, into the vitreous cavity (*tractional retinal detachment*).
- Exudation of material from the retinal vessels (such as in tumors, inflammations etc.) into the subretinal space (*exudative retinal detachment*).

The term *non-rhegmatogenous retinal detachment* refers collectively to the tractional and exudative retinal detachment.

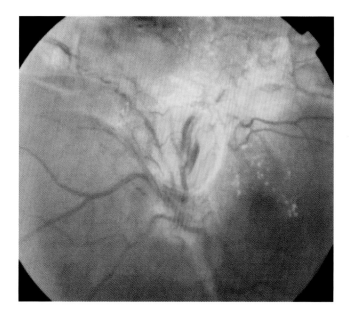

FIGURE 7.1: Tractional retinal detachment
Retinal detachment caused by pulling forward of the retina by the fibrovascular tissue

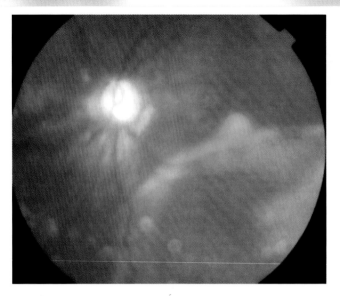

FIGURE 7.2: Retinal detachment
Longstanding inferior retinal detachment

In the case of rhegmatogenous retinal detachment, patients with high myopia (>6D) have a 5% risk, individuals with aphakia (without implant) have a 2% risk, and patients who had a vitreous loss during cataract operation, have a 10% risk. However, the incidence of retinal detachment following cataract surgery has greatly reduced with the use of phacoemulsification techniques because of small incision, maintenance of anterior chamber, posterior chamber implants, and lack of intraoperative complications. In patients of retinal detachment, nearly one-fifth of the fellow eyes develop a retinal detachment, later. Approximately 40-50% of all patients with retinal detachment are myopes, 30-40% are aphakic, and 10-20% have encountered direct ocular trauma.

Initial symptoms of retinal detachment commonly include the sensation of flashes (photopsia) along with floaters and reduced vision. The patient may complain of a shadow in a particular part of the visual field to begin with, the shadow gradually spreading to the entire visual field. Gross visual loss manifests in eyes where the retinal detachment includes the macula. In general, patients are less aware of a superior field defect (indicating an inferior detachment) than an inferior retinal detachment. Longstanding inferior detachments may be present without symptoms until the detachment progresses to involve the fovea *(Figure 7.2)*.

Fundus examination is made, under full mydriasis, with the indirect ophthalmoscope using scleral indentation. It may be supplemented, if required in some cases, by examination with a 3-mirror contact lens and scleral indentation. Obvious detachment appears as elevation of retina that looks gray *(Figure 7.3)*. Overlying blood vessels appear dark, and may lie in folds. Undulations of retina are seen in some eyes, during the course of funduscopy. The causative factor of the detachment is seen in the form of a hole, break or a tear *(Figure 7.4)* that may be of different size and shape. Frequently, such lesions are multiple. Concurrently, some form of peripheral retinal degeneration without a retinal tear, may also be present.

Treatment

Broad principles involved in the treatment of rhegmatogenous retinal detachment consist of cryo/laser coagulation of all the holes/tears in the retina; drainage of the fluid collected in the subretinal space; and neutralizing the traction on the retina. The release of traction may be achieved by way of scleral buckling, or

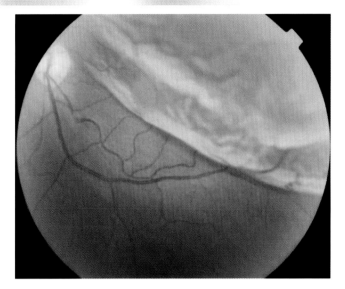

FIGURE 7.3: Retinal detachment
Gray looking, elevated retina with folds

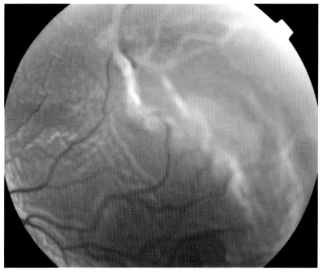

FIGURE 7.4: Retinal detachment
Flap tear in the 11 o'clock position deformed by a dense fold in the elevated retina; a number of small, irregular lines causing 'washerman skin' appearance resulting from the development of PVR

vitrectomy combined with membrane peeling, that is generally reserved for cases having proliferation of fibrous membranes on the anterior or posterior aspect of the retinal surface—*proliferative vitreo-retinopathy (PVR)*. Injection of vitreous substitutes like silicone oil, expandable gases, or fluid perfluorocarbons is reserved for cases of rhegmatogenous retinal detachment associated with severe form of PVR, and in most cases of secondary, tractional retinal detachment. *Retinotomy* and *retinectomy procedures* are required in certain complex situations.

Prophylaxis. Prophylactic treatment with regard to the indication and methodology has been a matter of conflicting opinions. Ideally, prophylactic treatment of retinal breaks can only be justified if the risk of complications from treatment is lower than the risk of breaks leading to retinal detachment. Unfortunately, no valid controlled studies have been made to reasonably settle the issue of risk-benefit ratio. Most of the current recommendations are based on the consensus.

Present evidence supports prophylactic treatment of all symptomatic retinal tears, large operculated retinal tears, retinal breaks with subclinical retinal detachment threatening progression, retinal tears before cataract surgery, retinal tears seen following the symptoms of acute posterior vitreous detachment (PVD), and high-risk fellow eyes of non-traumatic giant retinal tears. Asymptomatic retinal tears discovered in phakic eyes do not show any significant tendency towards clinical retinal detachment. Likewise, and contrary to the general belief, asymptomatic tears in aphakic or pseudophakic eyes, eyes with lattice degeneration *(Figure 7.5)*, high myopia, and fellow eye detachments show no subsequent benefit from prophylaxis and are to be followed without treatment.

Some reports have observed significantly reduced incidence of retinal detachment in the fellow eyes of cases with retinal detachment following prophylactic treatment of retinal breaks or lattice degeneration. A large, retrospective study, however, failed to make recommendations concerning what fellow eyes, if any, should undergo prophylactic treatment.

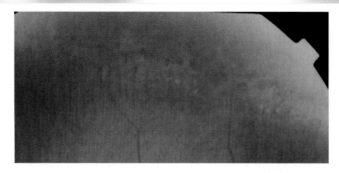

FIGURE 7.5: Retinal detachment
Lattice degeneration of the retina with atrophic retinal holes, located at the equatorial region

In another scenario, 360 degree laser photocoagulation of the retina anterior to the equator is strongly recommended in eyes subjected to vitrectomy for conditions like macular hole, tractional retinal detachments, trauma, etc.

Index

A

Acute multifocal
  choroiditis 85
  posterior pigment epitheliopathy (AMPPE) 83
Age-related macular degeneration (ARMD) 3
Angiographic features 7
Arterial occlusions 53
Astrocytoma 120
Avulsion of optic disk 115

B

Basal laminar drusen 2
Berlin's edema 50
Bests' disease 97
Branch retinal
  artery occlusion 53
  vein occlusion 65

C

Capillary hemangioma 118
Central areolar choroidal
  dystrophy 103
  sclerosis
Central retinal
  artery occlusion (CRAO) 53
  vein occlusion (CRVO) 58
Central serous retinopathy 22
Childhood optic neuritis 113
Choroidal
  folds 48
  neovascular membrane 44
  nevus 116
  rupture 48
Cilioretinal artery occlusion 57
Coats' disease 81
Combined CRAO-CRVO occlusion 57
Commotio retinae 50
Cone dystrophy 98
Congenital hypertrophy of retinal pigment epithelium (CHRPE) 117
Cystoid macular edema (CME) 36

D

Diabetic retinopathy 70
Disease of macula 1
Drusen 1
Dry type of ARMD 4

E

Eales' disease 90
Epimacular membrane (EMM) 51

F

Familial dominant drusen 103
Fundus
  flavimaculatus 96
  fluorescein angiography 53

G

Geographic helicoid peripapillary choroidopathy (GHPC) 86

H

Hard drusen 1
Hereditary diseases 96
Hypertensive retinopathy 68

I

Idiopathic
  juxtafoveolar retinal telangiectasia 41
  polypoidal choroidal vasculopathy 39
Inflammations 83
Ischemic CRVO 62

M

Macular
  hemorrahage 50
  hole 20
Melanocytoma 120
Myelinated nerve fibers 105
Myopic maculopathy 16

N

Non-ischemic CRVO 60
Non-proliferative diabetic retinopathy 73

O

Optic
  atrophy 113
  disk
    coloboma 106
    drusen 108
    pit 107
  nerve disorders 105
  neuritis 111

P

Papilledema 109
Parafoveal telangiectasia (PFT) 41
Periphlebitis retinae 90
Proliferative diabetic retinopathy (PDR) 76

R

Retinal
  detachment 121
  pigment epithelial detachment 34
  vascular diseases 53
Retinitis pigmentosa 99

S

Sarcoidosis 94
Soft drusen 2
Stargardt's macular dystrophy 96

T

Toxoplasmic retinochoroiditis 89
Tumors 116
Type of drusen 1

V

Venous occlusions 58
Vitelliform degeneration 97

W

Wet type of ARMD 6